THE PASSI
AND HARD

THE PASSIONATE LIVES OF DEAF AND HARD OF HEARING PEOPLE

Karen Putz

Barefoot Publications

Chicago, Illinois

CONTENTS

OTHER BOOKS BY KAREN PUTZ

Available on Amazon and Barnes and Noble:
Gliding Soles, Lessons from a Life on Water, co-authored with
Keith St. Onge
Barefoot Water Skiing, From Weekend Warrior to Competitor
The Parenting Journey, Raising Deaf and Hard of Hearing
Children
Dying to Tell (Coming soon)
Book cover designed by:
Leah Murray at Rochester Institute of Technology
Book edited by:
Lisa Florey

FOREWORD BY GLENN ANDERSON

Before I came to Gallaudet College (now University) in 1965, I had no clear idea of what was possible for me. What could I expect to do in the future? Since I was athletic and enjoyed playing sports, especially basketball, one of the career options I considered was becoming a Physical Education teacher and basketball coach.

At Gallaudet, I saw deaf people involved in jobs and leadership positions I had never envisioned were possible. They were working as administrators and faculty members. Gallaudet was also a place where deaf national organization leaders visited the campus as invited guest speakers. It was also the first time I became aware that deaf people were pursuing advanced degrees (at that time mostly at the Master's level). My eyes opened wide. What I had pictured for myself prior to my arrival at Gallaudet was limited. Deaf people were doing so much more and I realized I could do more too.

I eventually changed my major from Physical Education to Psychology, and after graduation I went to graduate school at the University of Arizona in 1968. Upon my arrival at the University of Arizona, my eyes were once again opened wide when I encountered deaf graduate students who were pursuing doctoral degrees. Prior to 1968, it was uncommon to hear of a deaf person pursuing a doctoral degree. Among the deaf doctoral students attending the University of Arizona at that time were several notables in the education and rehabilitation profession such as Victor Galloway, Larry Stewart, Richard Johnson, and Geno Vescovi. They each inspired me as role models and mentors and from time to time they hinted that I ought to consider going for my doctorate. But for me, the idea of a doctoral degree was the farthest thing from my mind. My immediate goal was to earn my master's degree, get a job, and enjoy life. But little did I know they had planted a seed in my mind and that one day later it would "bear fruit."

At the time I interviewed for my first professional job after graduate school, only a small number of deaf people worked as counselors in state vocational rehabilitation agencies throughout the nation. It meant that hearing agency managers responsible for interviewing and hiring deaf persons for professional positions, for the most part, had little, if any knowledge about what deaf people could or could not do as professional service providers. I also recall that I participated in the interview without the benefit of an interpreter. During my job interview, one of the first things the agency manager said to me was, "Our counselors are required to use the telephone to contact venders, employers, and clients. If you are not able to use the telephone, how are you going to be able to do the job?" At that time telephone relay services were not yet a reality. I was able to alleviate his concerns by mentioning how I could collaborate with an assistant or secretary to handle telephone calls.

During the early years of my professional career I recall hearing at national conferences that two of the often mentioned career-related obstacles for deaf people were: (1) their overrepresentation at the lower end of career ladder in jobs working as assembly line workers in factories and as clerks and baggage handlers for the Post Office and (2) limited opportunities to advance up the career ladder and break though "glass ceilings" to work in high-level management and leadership positions in the private and non-profit sectors.

Who could have predicted the sea change that would impact on the lives of deaf people in the late 1980s and thereafter? The success of the Deaf President Now (DPN) movement at Gallaudet University in 1988 created a paradigm shift with regard to how deaf people from that point forward viewed themselves as well as how hearing people viewed them. And along with major legislative and technological catalysts such as the enactment of the Americans with Disabilities Act and the explosive growth of computing, Internet, and video and telecommunications technology, many new opportunities opened up for deaf people. The opportunities that have opened up in the everyday lives for deaf people as our society progressed from the later part of the 20th century to the early onset of the 21st century are astounding.

So what are the possibilities for deaf people in the 21st century? What barriers are deaf people breaking down in today's job market? Who are the people marking their mark in our modern day society? What are their success stories? *The Passionate Lives of Deaf and Hard of Hearing People* shares revealing stories about deaf and hard of hearing people who are forging new paths of opportunity—many in areas that, for the most part, are considered unique and that are "eye-openers" as to what is possible for deaf people. The book's author, Karen Putz interviewed and profiled deaf and hard of hearing individuals from diverse professions and walks of life. Many of these individuals are what I would call "trailblazers" in that they dared to "dream big" and venture into uncharted territories for deaf and hard of hearing people. In the process of collecting their stories, Karen also noted that two commonalities possessed by her interviewees: passion and persistence. Each of the trailblazers discovered a passion for something that set their hearts on fire; and when the going got tough and they encountered "road blocks" to their paths, they did not give up and quit. They did not allow various obstacles that they encountered on the paths to deter their dreams.

Readers will find this book inspirational and informative as well as entertaining to read. For those considering their possibilities for the future, which at this time in our history offers almost limitless possibilities, the book aims to share a positive message:

with passion and persistence, deaf and hard of hearing people can do anything!

Glenn B. Anderson, Ph.D.

Department of Counseling, Adult, and Rehabilitation Education

University of Arkansas at Little Rock

Former Chair, Gallaudet University Board of Trustees, 1994-2005

INTRODUCTION BY KAREN PUTZ

Years ago, I was sitting across from a university guidance counselor trying to plan out my college courses and my future.

"I want to be a nurse," I said. "A labor and delivery nurse."

Gently, but firmly, the counselor discouraged my choice.

"The communication challenges would make it very difficult to do the job," the counselor explained. Shortly before arriving at the university, I lost my hearing after a hard fall while barefoot water skiing, progressing from hard of hearing to deaf. My self-esteem was in a shaky place at the time. I was struggling in my classes because I couldn't understand my teachers and I didn't know American Sign Language.

I tried to picture myself as a nurse, but the doubts began to take over.

How would I handle phone calls to the doctor if a mom's labor progressed? How would I understand a patient if their head was turned away from me? How could I possibly follow conversation in a room full of family members and hospital staff? What if my lack of hearing ability hurt a patient?

I didn't have the answer to those questions. Perhaps the counselor was right: The communication challenges were just too great. I dropped the career idea and looked for other careers to pursue. My mom suggested going into computers or accounting.

"You can get a good, solid job with those careers," she said. Yet, the idea of sitting in a cubicle day after day was not something I envisioned.

I thought back to high school. I loved writing. Poems, articles, book reports—writing came easy to me. At one point, I wanted to be a journalist. I pictured myself writing for a major newspaper or the magazines. My English teacher in high school encouraged me to write for the school newspaper. The news editor assigned me to do stories on different topics and sent me on all kinds of assignments. I struggled through them. I was assigned to do an article on the volleyball team and when I went to interview the volleyball coach, I missed a lot of what he said. The coach was very irritated when he had to repeat himself several times. I turned in a short, dismal article about the team. I cursed my hearing loss at every point of the experience. (And this was before I became deaf.)

After turning in the volleyball article, I was assigned to cover a school board meeting. Terror struck deep in the pit of my stomach. There was no way I could follow several people at once. Group conversations are the "Ping-Pong of Social Death" for a deaf or hard of hearing person. By the time you feast your eyes on one person talking, a second one has answered, and a third has chimed in.

Ironically, I was able to put together an article by obtaining a copy of the printed minutes a few days later. My journalism teacher declared it one of my best articles. Ever.

Well, yeah, I had full access to something solid to write with!

After reflecting on the limitations the guidance counselor set forth, I set aside the idea of a nursing career and contemplated something safe. Perhaps accounting would bring me a stable job with a good income, or something in the computer field, as my mom suggested. My heart just wasn't into either of those choices.

In the end, I settled for two counseling degrees with an emphasis on serving deaf and hard of hearing people. I enjoyed my job as a Deaf Services Coordinator and peer counselor but I longed to work with babies. To fill the void, I volunteered at a local hospital to care for newborn babies. I gave the babies their first baths shortly after birth and combed the vernix out of their matted hair. I spent hours rocking and feeding babies. There were some days when I had difficulty understanding some of the nurses, but for the most part, they were very accommodating.

The communication challenges reared their ugly head one day when a father came for his baby and I misunderstood the last name. He took one look at the baby I handed to him and said, "That's not my baby!" I quickly located the proper baby. My heart was pounding at the mistake. This was before the days of matching wristbands.

I met Randy, a hard of hearing nurse from the same hospital. Randy sported hearing aids and worked in the surgical unit. She had trained herself so well in the operating room that she knew what surgical instrument to hand the surgeon before they even asked for anything. After talking with Randy and being inspired by her, I decided to examine some careers I could pursue in a hospital setting.

I started exploring the idea of becoming an ultrasonographer. I figured it was a great way to be involved with babies without having to deal with too many communication barriers. I set up a day where I could shadow a technician at work with several patients. At the end of the day, I sat down with the director of nuclear medicine to ask every question I could think of about the job. When I left the hospital, I knew the ultrasound path was not for me. As much as I loved babies, I didn't want to spend all day measuring their body parts.

As the years unfolded, I met more and more deaf and hard of hearing people in the medical field. The first time I met Dr. Carolyn Stern, I was in awe. Profoundly deaf, she did not let a dean discourage her from pursuing her dream of becoming a doctor. She was doing her residency at Lutheran General Hospital near Chicago and she regaled me with stories of catching baby after baby. At that time, I was studying to be a doula and began attending home and hospital births. Becoming a doula was the perfect way for me to fulfill my passion of working with moms and babies.

By this time, more and more deaf and hard of hearing medical professionals began to pop up in my life. A veterinarian. A pharmacist. A dentist. A speech therapist. A nurse who worked in the ER. A school nurse. More doctors. Medical coders. Hospital managers. All them deaf or hard of hearing.

Can you imagine how different my state of mind might have been back in college if I had known about all the deaf and hard of hearing medical professionals out there?

Then one day, I received a call from a parent of a 15-year-old son. She called to ask some questions about jobs which would be a good fit for a hard of hearing kid. I was more interested in what her son wanted to do. *What were his skills? What were his passions? What were his dreams?*

"Well, he wants to be a doctor," she said. "But I know he can't do that."

"Yes, he can be a doctor if he wants to," I said.

There was *no way* this mom was going to get the same talk I received in college. So I told her about all the medical professionals I met over the years. The doctors. The nurses, The vets. The pharmacists. The dentists. The Association of Medical Professionals currently has over 200 deaf and hard of hearing professionals in their association. The estimate is probably far higher, I told her.

There was silence for a long time. I started to wonder if we had been disconnected. Then she spoke. She was full of questions. *What about stethoscopes?* They have amplified ones, I explained. *What about studying to become a doctor?* The schools can provide real-time captioning, I explained. *What about surgery?* Yes, there are doctors who do surgery using clear masks.

By the end of our phone call, the view of her son's future had totally changed. Her son's world had suddenly opened up with possibilities, instead of limits.

That's why I wrote this book.

This book is for every parent, every professional who works with deaf and hard of hearing people and every deaf and hard of hearing person who has a dream. I interviewed deaf and hard of hearing people from all different professions and life paths. There's a common theme among every single one of them: passion. Every one of them discovered a passion for something that set their heart on fire. They did not let the idea of being deaf or hard of hearing stop them.

Sure, there were challenges along the way and roadblocks on the path. Which leads me to another trait among these amazing guys and gals: persistence. Not one of them ever gave up, even when the going was tough or near impossible.

I tell people all the time—just because it hasn't been done before doesn't mean YOU or your child can't be the first to blaze the way. For every person who thinks in terms of barriers, there are others who are overcoming them and setting new heights. In the course of history, there has always been someone who walked an unknown path.

Today, maybe it will be you. Or your child. Go forth and blaze a passionate path.

Chapter 1

GREG GUNDERSON: RACING DREAMS

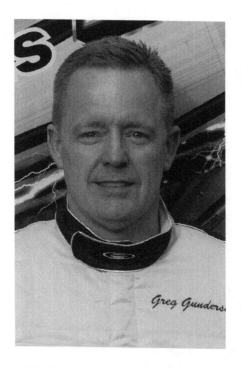

The racing bug bit Greg Gunderson when he was a baby, but he doesn't remember his first race. Greg's father arrived at a drag racing tournament with Greg in a car seat. He strapped Greg in, took off at the starting gate and won the race.

From the time he was a toddler, Greg spent his days sitting in a car in his father's garage watching his father and grandfather fine-tune the engine before every race.

"The car was my playground," Greg recalled. "When I was three, I was taking parts apart and putting them back together. I got all dirty in the process, but I loved it."

Greg was born deaf. His mother made this discovery after noticing that he was sleeping soundly as she vacuumed under his crib and a hearing test at the South Dakota School for the Deaf confirmed the diagnosis. Greg's father quickly called a deaf cousin and arranged for him to move in with the family so they could learn American Sign Language.

For Greg, his father, and his grandfather, the common language was racing. Greg went to every racing event with them. His father was a snowmobile dealer, so Greg went along to snowmobile races. One winter while his dad was off talking with others, six-year-old Greg signed himself up in the youth division. Most of the kids were eight and older. He grabbed his father's snowmobile and went over to the starting line. The machine was a little big for him to handle, but the moment the flag dropped, Greg gunned for the finish line.

Later that night at the awards dinner, Greg's name was announced as the first-place winner for the kid's division. Of course, Greg didn't hear his name called. His father turned to him in surprise and said, "They announced your name–there must be a mistake!"

Greg smiled with pride.

"I won the race!" he signed. His father stared at him in shock. His six-year-old deaf son had just beaten a bunch of kids who were older than him. Greg took home a check for $200.

Back home on the farm, despite being an only child, life was fun. Greg had motocross and snowmobile tracks in his backyard. After school, he would hit the tracks and race with his Uncle Guy, who was 14 years older.

"Every day, I would arrive home tired but when I got to the track, I would ride and ride. That was my medicine," Greg said. He did various races: ATVs, motocross, and dirt bikes. On the weekends, Greg and a friend would head to his grandparent's lake house and water ski.

In his junior year of high school, Greg and a friend went to a local race one weekend. Greg shelled out a dollar on a raffle ticket and settled in his seat to watch the race. During intermission, they announced his name as the winner of an Enduro race car. Greg was in shock when they handed him the keys. The following week, he entered his first entry-level race.

"I was really nervous and breathing too fast–I fogged up my helmet," Greg said. "I had to push up the visor so I could see."

Six races later, Greg was in the turn when the car behind bumped him, sending him into the wall and head-on into another car. Greg walked away unscathed, but the car was totaled.

Greg couldn't let go of the racing bug.

"I want to race sprint cars!" he told his grandfather. A deaf sprint car driver? His grandfather couldn't see it happening.

"No, it's too fast and dangerous," his grandfather warned.

But Greg didn't give up the vision. The summer after he graduated from high school, Greg hung out with a sprint car team. He offered to work for them and would do anything for the chance to drive a car.

"The night before I was to leave for Gallaudet, they let me drive the car during intermission," Greg said. "I did eight laps. It was like a drug for me. I couldn't let go of racing after that moment."

During the summer break, Greg spied a race car in a friend's garage. His friend couldn't afford to put an engine in the car. Every single day, Greg stopped by the house to convince his friend to let him fix up the car and race it. Finally in July, his friend gave in and said, "Take the car!"

Greg was grinning from ear to ear when he towed the car on a trailer to his uncle's garage.

But Greg had a dilemma, he didn't have any money for an engine. How was he going to get the car ready for a race?

There was one thing Greg did have a lot of: determination. Greg scouted several people who could help him put together an engine and the equipment he needed to race. Pretty soon, he had an engine, a race suit, and everything he needed to enter his first sprint car race.

"I paid not one cent on that car," Greg chuckled.

Before the race, Greg contacted the race officials and arranged to do some practice runs. And when he crossed the finish line at his first sprint car race, he landed in fourth place, outperforming some veterans who had been racing for years.

"After that race, they all finally realized, 'Hey, I can race!'" Greg said. He raced a couple more times that summer and went back to college.

During Christmas break, his friend sold the car. Greg was back to square one. But he did it once before, he could do it again. Greg rounded up the parts for another car and his Uncle Guy agreed to work on it, sending Greg pictures of the progress. By the summer, Greg was back in the seat racing again. Despite a much smaller engine than the other cars, Greg landed in the top five or 10 in every race. But he soon realized he would never be able to compete at the top until he had a better car.

Another friend stepped forward. Ron Tysdal purchased a car for Greg and he soon won his first heat. Then five more in a row.

At the Sioux Empire Fair in his hometown of Sioux Falls, South Dakota, Greg did poorly in a race one Friday night.

"My grandfather and Ron told me not to go back and race the next day," Greg said. "But my Uncle Guy encouraged me to go without telling them, so I did."

Greg made it all the way to the finals.

"I lined up at the starting pole and I took off in the lead," Greg recalled. "I didn't know how much of a lead, but around and around we went until the white flag went up, which means one more lap left. I was excited–I was in the lead. The last lap took forever!"

As soon as the black and white checkered flag dropped, Greg realized he had won. It was a sweet victory against so many experienced drivers. The announcer explained to the crowd that Greg was deaf. During his celebration lap, fans in the stand didn't clap–they stood up and waved their hands in the air. TV reporters and radio personalities swarmed him to get the story. With the help of pen and paper and his uncle interpreting, Greg answered their questions.

"Without a doubt, this race is one which stands out in my mind the most, because it was my first major win," Greg said. "But the following week, I was overconfident. I was in front, but on the 10th lap I was too fast. I lost control, flipped over, and destroyed the car. I went from hero to zero!"

Greg has won many more races since then. He has done more than 750 races and has no plans to stop anytime soon. In fact, he's got an even bigger dream on the horizon: NASCAR. At first glance, that almost seems impossible, but Greg has tested out new technology with an innovative company using a car that would enable him to communicate with a pit crew. It can be done; it will just take a sponsor who has the same vision to make it happen.

For more information about Greg and his racing career, visit www.gundersonracing.com.

CHAPTER 2

AMY DUARTE: ANIMATING HOLLYWOOD MOVIES

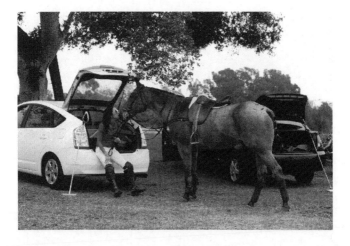

Amy Duarte was just five years old when she figured out what she wanted to do in life. She was deep into watching the lively animation of Cinderella dancing on the TV when she told her parents, "That's what I want to do!"

While most little girls dreamed of becoming Cinderella and dancing around in a ball gown, Amy wanted to be the person who made Cinderella come to life on the screen. For 11 years, Amy trained in classical ballet.

"To me, it was a form of training, discipline, and it required a lot of physical hard work. Come on, wearing a tutu and dancing on toes qualifies as a sport, doesn't it?" she said grinning.

Amy attended California State University at Northridge and landed an internship with the Walt Disney Company. Her dream of animating major movies came true: the internship turned into a full-time job as a visual effects artist.

A typical day for Amy begins with a client conference call or meeting with as many as 30 people. On some projects, Amy meets with the team in a dark screening room and reviews the shots on a large screen or she conducts a call at her desk while doing interactive shot reviews on the computer.

"During the conference call, I would get notes pertaining to the shots from the client," Amy explained. "For example, in one of my shots, Spiderman's visor is too dark, he needs better motion blur as he's swinging across the city, and we need heavier atmosphere for the cityscape. I address those issues right after the meeting, spend the next few hours making a new iteration, and then submit the new version for the afternoon conference call. The whole cycle repeats until the shot is finalized and approved."

During the production for the movie *Fantastic Four*, Amy was promoted to sequence lead artist and supervised her team on lighting effects for the movie. If an artist was lagging behind, Amy jumped in and took over the shots.

"It was such an honor to be entrusted with such a responsibility," Amy said. "By the end of the show, my supervisor became one of my very good friends in the industry. We continued to collaborate on other projects. It is a wonderful feeling knowing that I have earned someone's trust–especially someone of that stature and position."

Amy has another passion that qualifies as a sport: polo. She grew up riding horses, competing in dressage/horse jumping events since she was six.

"When I was 14, I saw a video of a polo match and I wanted to try it," Amy said. "Back then, I did not know how to get into polo or where to go for that. I was under the impression that polo was for people like Prince Charles and ladies with big hats sipping champagne, going 'Hee hee, hoo hoo.'"

Amy discovered the California Polo Club in Los Angeles and she signed up for her first lesson. The early lessons were challenging.

"I kept missing the ball in the first few lessons. It got to the point where the horse sighed at me in exasperation," Amy laughed. "I am not joking, it actually happened! I guess it was the horse's way of calling me an idiot."

As a deaf player, Amy has to be visually aware of what's happening on the field to compensate for what she can't hear while galloping on a horse at 35 mph. Her teammates work together to let her know when the bell rings to signal the end of a game.

"It's a challenge to hear what's going on in the heat of the battle, because when my teammates are yelling, 'Go for the pass, Amy!' or 'The ball is right under you, Amy!' I don't have the luxury of asking politely, 'Pardon me, what did you say?'" Amy said.

Amy fell in love with polo, and the next step was to determine how to afford her own horse. She sat down with a financial adviser and mapped out a plan to make it work. After some dedication and sacrifice, Amy purchased her first polo horse.

"It's the beauty of the relationship between man and horse. You are putting your life into the hands of this 1,500-pound beast while galloping at 35 mph. I've seen polo players reach so far out to the right (or left) to hit the ball with the horse still running in a straight line. That requires a lot of faith and trust in the animal carrying you. I've muttered so many 'Hail Marys' while playing this sport. I just pray to come out alive and in one piece. I guess another part of the attraction of this sport is the adrenaline rush!"

It's easy to see how hard work, determination, and goals are what has propelled Amy forward in every area of her life. She

unwrapped her dream of being an artist at an early age and she def-
initely did not let anything stand in her way.

"There is no substitute for hard work," Amy said. She shares
more:

> I knew from my early childhood years that I wanted to work as an artist
> for the film industry. I took the necessary classes and training to further
> advance my skills. Many hours were spent building my portfolio and demo
> reel. I took full advantage of a wonderful internship at Walt Disney Stu-
> dios—I'd come in early and stay late to put extra effort in whatever I was
> doing—and I'd ask for constructive criticism for my artwork. That way, I
> built relationships and rapport. In turn, that opened up doors when other
> opportunities came along. My point is, we all have to keep working at it.
> What amazes me is when a deaf person tells me it's a lot easier just to live
> off disability checks because 'Life is too hard being deaf.' I ask them, 'Have
> you really put in your 100 percent effort into it? Have you done enough
> research on what it takes to accomplish your goals?' More often than not,
> they'll admit that they didn't put in their full effort or they think that some
> jobs were beneath them. I remind them that I started on the bottom too.
> My jobs were not always glamorous—I started with nothing and worked
> my way up.

"Again, let me repeat," Amy said. "There's no substitute for hard
work."

CHAPTER 3

BRENDA STOLTZ: CEO OF ARIAD PARTNERS

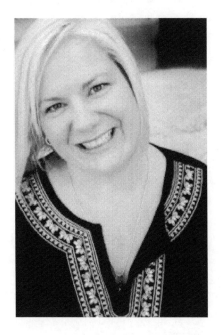

Brenda Stoltz was raised all over the country, moving from state to state as her father changed jobs. As a child who grew up hard of hearing, Brenda quickly learned to adapt.

"From an early age, I learned how to talk to a lot of different people," Brenda said. "This served me well later in my business."

Brenda grew up with a progressive hearing loss and her family treated it as if the problem did not exist. Brenda shared some of her experience:

The tough part was I never really felt accepted–I felt very different. I knew no one else that was deaf or hard of hearing, and my parents didn't look for other people in the deaf or hard of hearing community to socialize with. They certainly never considered that I needed to learn American Sign Language, so I felt isolated in that respect. We never talked about it–it was hard. There was a silver lining though–I was forced to adapt and depend on myself. The burden was on me to communicate; to watch and lipread. I became exceptionally good at lipreading and I learned to communicate effectively. My parents today will still talk behind my back as if I could hear them! I have to get in front of them and remind them to look at me. In a way, that's real life, that's the world around us. I had to adapt and it made me stronger for that. It was hard growing up, but then again, it's hard no matter what.

Brenda became deaf when she was a young adult.

"I would notice when I would lose sound–I could hear the phone ring one day and then the next day, I couldn't hear it," Brenda said. "I could hear the birds, and then one day, I couldn't hear them anymore. It was a slow progression."

During a visit to an audiologist, she contemplated leaving her hearing aids out and living her life without them. At that point, she could not hear critical speech sounds and could only hear low tones. With her hearing aids, she could hear some environmental sounds; without them, not much of anything.

The audiologist asked, "How many deaf people do you see every day?"

"None," Brenda replied.

"I still remember the audiologist's response. She said, 'You will make more money and have a better quality of life if you keep the hearing aids on and live in the hearing world,'" Brenda said.

Since she was raised orally, Brenda didn't know sign language and she didn't know anyone who was deaf, but she was interested in learning more. It was an interesting time in her life filled with lots of questions. She was lucky enough to have a neighbor who was an interpreter and this neighbor introduced her to others who were deaf.

"My first experience with the deaf community wasn't good," Brenda said. "They didn't want to interact with me. I didn't sign. I didn't know their language and I didn't feel welcome. I was caught between two worlds in those days. Luckily, today there is a lot more openness in the hearing and deaf communities, and I've met so many people in both who are much more understanding."

College was a nightmare at first. When Brenda walked into her first class, she encountered a teacher with an accent, a full beard, and a penchant for using the board while talking.

"Lipreading was impossible, and I had no idea that any support services might have been available for me," Brenda said. She studied hard, persevered, and graduated with a double major in business and humanities.

At one of her first jobs, Brenda worked at a bank as a receptionist.

"I told the interviewer I wanted the job. I was a hard worker, but I couldn't hear on the phone. I worked for the vice president at the bank. I would get calls and take the name and the number–and never get them right–I got them wrong all the time."

Despite the rough start on the job, Brenda moved to a different position in finances and received several promotions. She continued to learn. Whatever skill was needed, Brenda expressed a positive attitude and worked to learn the skills necessary to do the job well.

"I pushed myself," she explained. "I knew I could learn the job and excel at it–I knew that in my heart."

At that time, Brenda was traveling all over the world for her job as a product manager in Silicon Valley. While working in San Francisco, Brenda met and fell in love with her future husband, Ken Stoltz. She did what she could to hide the progressive loss of hearing, but one day Ken called her on it and told her she needed to stop hiding it.

"He changed how I see myself," Brenda said. "He's the one who said, 'Brenda, you are deaf and you need to tell people this, make them aware, and let them know they need to be responsible for the communication as well. Telling people you're hard of hearing, that's not enough; it's not working for you. You need to own it.'"

Little by little, from that point on, Brenda became comfortable with being deaf and began to share her experience with others.

Brenda and Ken have two daughters, one who is also deaf. After staying home with her daughters for a few years, Brenda found herself itching to work again so she formed a consulting business, Ariad Partners, which serves mid-size businesses.

"Ariad is a play on the name of a Princess Ariadne of Greek mythology. She gave Theseus the tools he needed to find his way through the Minotaur's Labyrinth," Brenda explained. "Likewise, Ariad Partners was founded to provide the tools to lead businesses through the maze of the modern business environment."

Brenda also teaches classes in social media, business, and marketing at Northern Virginia Community College. Brenda absolutely loves her work and she works for altruistic reasons: she loves helping others and solving problems within businesses. In fact, on most days she finds it difficult to push herself away from the desk, but she sticks to a strict schedule to keep a harmonious balance in her life. Fridays, weekends, and evenings are devoted to family time.

As for her deaf daughter, Brenda wants to make sure she realizes that the whole world is open to her.

"She can do anything, the world is hers," Brenda said. "I taught her that everyone is different–some wear glasses, some wear hearing aids, some are in wheelchairs...if someone looks perfect, they're not. I want her to know that everyone has something that makes them feel different–if they look perfect, on the inside maybe they feel differently. We can't always see what differences people have."

As for Ariad Partners, Brenda sees herself doing this for years to come. She works with a core team of five or six contractors and occasionally pulls more on to her team for bigger clients.

"I'm very appreciative and grateful for my life, it's a good life. I'm happy. I have a great family, a great husband and kids–there's no lack of anything in my life because I'm deaf."

Find out more about Brenda's business at www.ariadpartners.com.

CHAPTER 4

I. KING JORDAN: GOING THE EXTRA MILE

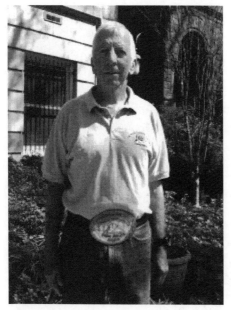

I. King Jordan is known for becoming the first deaf president of Gallaudet University in 1988, but there is a whole other side to King: the ultramarathoner. King regularly endures marathons of 50 to 100 miles and even endurance marathons consisting of 36 hours of running.

King joined the Navy right after high school and served four years. When he was 21, he crashed his motorcycle and landed head-first in the windshield of a car, fracturing his skull. When he woke up in the hospital, he discovered he was deaf. He was discharged from the Navy and began a new journey at Gallaudet University as a student.

King's passion for running began after he sprained his ankle in a basketball game and took up running to keep active. He discovered he had a talent for long-distance running.

"When I first started running, I began with 10-mile races and then moved on to 26.2-mile marathons," King said. "When I learned about ultramarathons, I was intrigued. I ran in 50-mile marathons and then I decided to try my first 100-mile marathon at Leadville."

The Leadville 100 "Race Across the Sky" is an annual race held in the Rocky Mountains of Colorado. The ultramarathon consists of running 100 miles on rocky terrain and narrow trails from an elevation of 9,200 to 12,600 feet. King ran the Leadville 100 year after year. During the 87th mile of his 10th Leadville, it was raining and King was running downhill when he slipped and fell.

"I hurt my back and I was in so much pain," King recalled. "That was my first DNF (did not finish) race and it was my 10th Leadville. When you finish 10 in Leadville, you get a gold belt buckle. The committee had already made my buckle with my name on it, but couldn't give it to me. I had my family and friends there to celebrate, but I couldn't celebrate. It was a good thing actually. It made me appreciate and understand others who had dropped out. Now I understand there are times when you can't finish."

The following year, King ran the Leadville again and he was determined to claim the belt buckle. King's wife, Linda, greeted him every 10 miles and handed him pop and Gatorade to keep him going.

"I needed the sugar to keep going and the pop to keep me awake," King explained. One hundred miles later, King wore the coveted buckle around his waist.

King has done three marathons where he has run for 36 hours straight. Running in the darkness is a challenge for him, because he has poor vestibular balance in the dark.

"If a hearing person trips, then his vestibular system will help regain balance, but if I trip, I usually end up on the ground with cuts and bruises. I know I'm going to fall when I run in the dark and people tell me, 'You can't do that' and I say 'To the heck with that, I sure can.'

"I hate extolling limits," King continued. "Some of my running success comes from proving what I could do. It really hurts to go on for hours and hours."

Speaking of success, King noticed a common trend among students during his years at Gallaudet. He noticed that many of the international students were graduating with high grades and going on to gainful employment. The international students often had to work hard and struggle just to get into Gallaudet—they were grateful for the opportunity and put in the work. King noticed some students who were afforded a lot of privilege and opportunities had a much more casual attitude about hard work and the results showed in their grades and lack of success.

"The ones who succeed at life are the ones who work—it's so straightforward and simple," King said. "Successful people put their nose to the grindstone."

King has some advice to share with parents of deaf and hard of hearing children: "Don't impose limits, because if you suggest limits to your child, that child will have limits," King explained. "If you believe they can't do things, then they won't. If you tell them again and again there are no limits, you can inspire your child to do anything they want."

CHAPTER 5

MELODY AND RUSS STEIN: A RESTAURANT DREAM BECOMES A REALITY

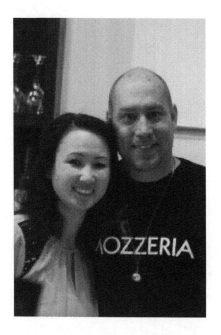

Tucked into a 100-year-old building in the heart of San Francisco is Mozzeria, a restaurant where every server knows American Sign Language and they dish up some heart-warming plates such as pizza topped with truffle honey and candied almond.

Mozzeria is owned by Melody and Russ Stein. Melody was

born in Hong Kong and went to school in the Philippines until her family moved to the United States so she could attend the California School for the Deaf at Fremont at the age of six. Her father had always owned restaurants around the world and when he opened a Chinese restaurant in San Francisco several years later, Melody started dreaming of someday owning her own restaurant.

Russ grew up in a deaf family. He spent his early years in classrooms with deaf students, but once the family moved to Florida, Russ and his deaf brother spent their days in the classroom without interpreters. Russ struggled day after day to understand everything being said.

"I had to do more than the other students, I had to work harder," Russ said. "I was always the teacher's favorite–I showed up, I sat and I never challenged my teachers–never raised my hand. I came up to my teachers after every class and asked, 'Did you say this or this?' to make sure I was getting the information right.

"I spent my life struggling to get communication–I bluffed a lot," Russ continued. "When I went to Gallaudet, it was heaven. I could understand all the conversations around me and I didn't have to struggle. I became a leader instead of a follower."

Melody started studying restaurant hospitality and management at the Rochester Institute of Technology, but the transition was a bit of a shock for her at first–she was not used to using interpreters all day in every class. Two years later, she transferred to Gallaudet, where she met Russ. After two years at Gallaudet, Melody decided to transfer to San Francisco State University to finish her degree in hospitality management.

"At that time, I saw an article about a struggling restaurant which was running an essay contest," Melody said. "The winner would win the restaurant space for free. So I wrote an essay based on Martin Luther King's 'I Have a Dream' speech, because I had a dream, too."

Unfortunately, the contest was dropped. Melody's dream would have to wait a bit longer.

A year later, the couple moved to Sioux Falls, South Dakota, where Russ became one of four people who fathered the start of Video Relay Services at the Communication Services for the Deaf. For 10 years they were content, but Russ was challenged with health issues and diagnosed with Crohn's disease. They transferred to Austin, Texas, to take advantage of the warmer climate. Melody was working in marketing and began to tire of the constant traveling. By this time, two children had joined the mix and Melody's parents often came in to take care of the kids when she was on the road. During one of their visits, her parents suggested a move back to San Francisco so they could provide child care on a regular basis. The arrangement worked well for a year. Melody continued her marketing job and Russ turned to consulting work while continuing to recover from his health issues.

The idea of owning a restaurant only grew stronger in their minds.

"I was done with traveling and I really wanted to be with my kids," Melody said. "It takes a lot of money to open a restaurant and we had a lot of hospital bills, so we decided to start small with a frozen yogurt business."

The idea got off to a rocky start when the couple couldn't agree on a name for the business. Then Russ had an idea: Why not start a pizza business instead? Russ enjoyed New York-style pizza from his years of growing up in New York, but Melody wasn't too crazy about the idea. To her, pizza equated fast food, and that was not the kind of restaurant she envisioned.

One night, the two of them dined at a restaurant that served a Neapolitan-style pizza. Melody peppered the waitress with questions and learned the pizza was developed in southern Italy and cooked in special ovens. As soon as they arrived home, Melody hopped on the computer and began to research pizzas. Just two weeks later, she was on a plane to Naples, Italy, with her mother. They spent 10 days learning everything they could about the Italian way of making pizzas and sauce.

Back home, Melody and Russ experimented with every aspect of pizza-making. Russ built an outdoor pizza oven in their backyard and they tested recipe after recipe, hosting "tasting parties" with their friends, and recording their feedback. They drew up a business plan and set out to obtain financing from local banks.

"The banks gave us a hard time," Melody said. "Every time I submitted the business proposal, they would turn it down and they didn't even read it. We were turned down so many times that we began to think it would be impossible to secure financing."

Russ and Melody turned to private investors and finally obtained the funding they needed and located a building to rent. They faced challenge after challenge while renovating the space for the restaurant, having to reinforce the floor for the wood-burning oven and run an insulated pipe up through several floors and out the roof. All of the renovations, with one exception, were completed by deaf-owned businesses. The majority of the staff are deaf, including the waiters.

Mozzeria opened during the holiday season and took off right from the start.

"On the opening night, the hearing customers were not used to our deaf staff," Melody said. "We have now served over 35,000 customers and counting—they keep coming back for the high-quality food we serve. Ironically, we also get compliments on our background music, which our hearing servers pick out for us."

Technology has made it easy to set up reservations online. The restaurant was so busy that Melody and Russ had no time to shop for Christmas gifts for their family.

"Now I realize how hard it to own a business and how challenging it is, whether you're deaf or hearing," Russ said. "I learned a lot from my dad. He owned a watch repair business and taught me to have patience. He taught me not to worry about the small things—if you experience big challenges, then you ignore the little things—you appreciate things differently. My dad also taught me

that life is not fair–it's what you do about it that makes a difference."

Today, the restaurant is thriving and they consistently receive
high reviews for their food and service. The couple are often contacted by others who are interested in learning how they can run
their own businesses.

Melody has some advice to share: "You have to believe in yourself– passion will see you to the finish line, it will carry you."

For more information about the restaurant, visit
www.mozzeria.com.

Chapter 6

HEIDI ZIMMER: CLIMBING NEW HEIGHTS

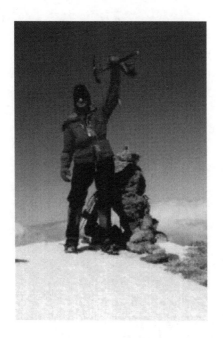

As a kid, Heidi Zimmer loved to climb. One day, Heidi's mom searched everywhere in the house for the two-year-old toddler but could not find her. She walked outside and found the two-year-old perched on the roof of their 1950s bungalow.

"My mother was scared, she ran next door to my father's office, where he worked as a pastor," Heidi said. "Ironically, my father is scared of heights, so a member of the church climbed up to get me. I don't remember how I got up on the roof, but that was the start of my passion for climbing."

Heidi's quest for exploration continued to blossom and she would spend hours and hours wandering through the towns around her. During college, she signed up for an Outward Bound trip that changed her life. The instructor could sign and one of the eight students was hard of hearing. Heidi found herself frustrated at the team's progress on the first day and walked off on her own.

"I quickly learned a lesson," Heidi said. "I could have gotten hurt walking alone in the wilderness. My survival depended on staying with my team."

For 23 days, the girls lived in the mountains, conserving water and surviving with the bare minimum. During a conversational moment with her instructor, Heidi shared her dream of climbing Mount Everest.

"Do you think I can do it?" she asked.

"Why not? Go for it!" her instructor said.

The response lifted Heidi's spirit–she had never received such positive encouragement like that before. Deaf or not, someone believed in her.

"When I flew back to college, I felt spoiled by the whole experience," Heidi said. "Living in the mountains changed my perspective on life. Before the trip, I was hooked on texting, but after 23 days in the wilderness I learned to let go of technology. Statistics show that the Outward Bound program increases self-esteem."

After graduating from Gallaudet, Heidi worked in the aerospace industry. The mountains continued to call out to Heidi so she started planning for her first climb. She selected Denali in Alaska as the first summit to conquer. It took 17 days to reach the 20,320 foot summit–the group was snowed in for four days nearly at the top. Two days later, during the descent, Heidi had a scary moment when she stepped into a crevasse (a deep crack in the ice) and went over the edge. She quickly regained her balance and scrambled back on the path.

"When I'm climbing and I'm frustrated…I just have to figure it out," Heidi said. "I learn from making mistakes, and when you make mistakes, you grow. You learn from mistakes. You have to be willing to do things you're not comfortable with to achieve great things.

"For example, I'm with hearing people 24/7 when I climb, and I'm not comfortable, but I do it. I have to do it to get to the top."

While climbing Kilimanjaro, Heidi discovered she was one of the few who spoke English. This put all the climbers on the same level in communicating with each other in different languages.

"When hearing people go into another country with different languages, they become 'deaf'–the communication challenges are all the same!"

Heidi was the first deaf woman to climb Denali and Mount Kilimanjaro, and the first deaf person to climb Mount Elbrus. She aims to be the first deaf person to reach all seven of the world's highest summits. For Heidi, mountain climbing is her passion and she plans to climb her way into the Highpoints Club by reaching the highest peak in every state. She has eight more states to go.

"Where others have chosen a traditional path, there's a question of 'should I follow and do the right thing.' I choose to spend my time and money in the mountains," Heidi explained. "People often think they must have a house, money, and a good job–but they don't live–they don't have a life. I follow my passion and I'm happy.

"The important thing is to follow what's in your heart. You don't have to follow the status quo. Break tradition! I'm not a follower. It's like a triangle paradigm: On the bottom, many do the same thing, and at the top are the rare few who are different."

The challenges of climbing mountains have taught Heidi how to handle the challenges of life. Heidi was diagnosed with Usher syndrome and has low vision due to retinitis pigmentosa. She battled breast cancer.

"It's a stumble on the journey," Heidi said. "I've faced many challenges–born deaf, Usher syndrome, and now breast cancer. Whatever it is, I face it. My father once said to me, 'Remember this: It's not what you face, but how you face it that counts.'"

For more information on Heidi and to follow her climbing endeavors, visit www.heidizimmer.com.

Chapter 7

JONATHAN NICOLL: NATURAL BODYBUILDING

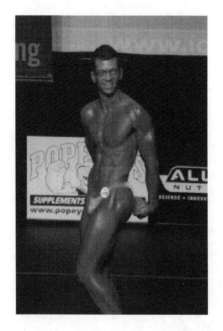

Jonathan Nicoll grew up in a small, rural area of Ontario, Canada. His parents owned a business renovating homes and as an only child, Jonathan played by himself while his parents worked.

"One day, my father made a loud noise in the same room that I was sitting in. My back was turned and I didn't respond," Jonathan said. The five year old was diagnosed with a moderate hearing loss and he started school in a program with other deaf and hard of hearing students. A year later, Jonathan moved to his local school with no support services until fifth grade. From fifth grade until high school, he spent 30 minutes per day with an itinerant teacher focusing on reading, writing, and life skills such as using the telephone. He valued his teacher so much he arrived a half hour early each day before heading to his high school classes.

"In high school, I was the only deaf student," Jonathan said. "One hard of hearing student dropped out and two others moved away. I had acquaintances whom I hung out with, but I was really shy and not confident. I couldn't join in their conversations–it was lonely. I followed whatever they wanted to do, because I didn't want to be alone. I didn't understand the concept of true friend-ships."

Keeping up in his classes was no easy feat. The communication challenges were tough.

"I didn't have confidence to share my thoughts–dialogue in the classroom was fast and I was too busy trying to follow everything what they said, and moving my head back and forth to follow the conversation. I would have to turn to see what was being said," Jonathan recalled.

During a session with the itinerant teacher, Jonathan shared his struggles and concerns about his future.

"I confessed that I didn't think I could graduate from universi-ty," Jonathan said. "She said, 'Yes, you can.' She changed my world during high school. She also advised me that high school sucks for most kids. I felt like there was no one else like me among 1,800 stu-dents. My teacher told me to focus on doing well, and assured me life would be better after high school."

When Jonathan sat down with the school guidance counselor to talk about going to university, he was met with some resistance at first.

"I don't know if you're ready for university," she told him.

Yet, when she pulled up his grades, she expressed some surprise: Jonathan had racked up some high marks in his classes. He went on to graduate from Queen's University and pursued his dream of becoming a teacher.

"Today, I'm a teacher for the deaf and I work at one of the four schools for the deaf in Ontario. I teach one high school class, one elementary, and a lot of one on one," Jonathan said.

Jonathan's journey into natural bodybuilding began as a youngster. Back when he was eight years old, Jonathan stumbled across a bodybuilding magazine and convinced his father to buy it for him. He was fascinated by the process of building muscles and sculpting bodies. In high school, he spent a little time in the weightlifting room. He discovered a weightlifting class on the school calendar, but was too shy to sign up for it.

One day, while surfing the Internet, Jonathan came across Nate Green's blog, *From Scrawny to Brawny*. Intrigued, Jonathan began to read more and more about natural bodybuilding and grabbed a copy of Nate's book. He signed up at a local gym and began to walk there and work out in the mornings. He began to connect with people in the natural bodybuilding network and found himself a coach and mentor to learn from.

"What's your dream?" the coach asked Jonathan. Jonathan was reluctant to share his dream at first, but his coach persisted.

"I want to enter a natural bodybuilding competition," Jonathan finally confessed.

"What are you waiting for?" his coach prodded.

Jonathan wasn't sure he was ready to take the leap, but he began preparing for competition. He had five months to work out and get ready. He found a more experienced coach from another state and communicated via emails and texts, sending him pictures of his progress.

"I had to learn everything at once: how to pose properly, prepare my body, and wear a suit with confidence," Jonathan said. "The biggest challenge I faced was I could not visualize myself on the stage. I practiced it, and in the last two weeks, I could finally see myself on stage. That whole process was an opportunity to really believe in myself. Many people believed in me, but I didn't believe in myself–they were great with their support."

The competition ended up being a life-changing event for Jonathan. Despite being way out of his comfort zone, he walked on stage and flexed his poses. Out of seven contestants, he placed sixth, but the placement didn't matter; the confidence he gained from that experience was priceless.

"Even if I came in last, it would have been fine," Jonathan said. "I was breaking all of my barriers–it was not about the medals or the trophy. I don't have any more fears or obstacles. I realized I can do whatever I want. I'm filled with confidence now. I know if I want to go and aim for something, I can."

Jonathan shared more:

Where I am today–it wouldn't be possible without all the other people who helped me get where I am today. The coaches helped me learn to believe in myself. My coaches believed in me. All the people on my 'team' helped me to realize that I wasn't alone. It doesn't matter if you're hard of hearing, deaf, or hearing–someone will show up in their life and help them realize themselves. I didn't like myself until I was 28–now I'm 31. I remember the day I really loved myself for the first time–my perspective of myself changed. The biggest change in me was this: I had been thinking negatively for many years and I changed to thinking positively. It's like that quote from Gandhi, 'Be the change you wish to see in the world.' That quote made me realize I had to change for my own happiness, my own life, my own dreams. I couldn't rely on other people to do that for me. I waited for that for 28 years. Once I took the responsibility for my own happiness, I became happier. Weightlifting taught me this and I apply it to my job, my friendships, everything. Weightlifting was my teacher for life.

Today, Jonathan is reaching out and sharing his life lessons with others.

"I attended the Canadian Hard of Hearing Association-International Federation of Hard of Hearing Congress in Vancouver for the first time," Jonathan said. "Among the nuggets of wisdom that I learned was Adam Ungstad's line, 'One's comfort zone is one's disability.' I heard from Monique Les, 'It's not about how much hearing you have; it's about what you do with the hearing that you have,' and I learned from Cai Glover's experience while performing as a ballet dancer.

"I came back home seeing myself through a new lens: I am a person first and someone who has many interests and dreams, and who happens to be hard of hearing. For the first time ever, I learned that I am not my hearing loss."

CHAPTER 8

JOEL BARISH: TRAVELING THE WORLD

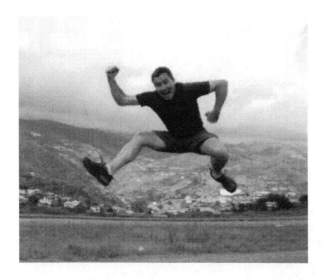

A huge map of the world hangs on one wall in Joel Barish's office. Joel has made a career out of traveling around the globe. He captures the stories of deaf and hard of hearing folks from all walks of life. Along with his brother Jed, Joel is best known for running DeafNation, a series of trade shows in the United States that is now expanding around the world.

Joel graduated from Gallaudet University with a degree in TV/

film production. His goal was to work for a major studio and produce films.

"Filming wasn't easy," Joel recalled. "The equipment was heavy and nothing like today's cameras. We didn't have digital back then."

After college, Joel took a detour in his career path, opening a travel agency and a coffee shop. This was back in the days before Starbucks was born. At the time, he was one of only two deaf travel agents. For three years, he managed the agency/coffee shop, then decided to close the business and take a job with American Express Travel Service.

Dr. Donalda Ammons, Joel's Spanish teacher at Gallaudet, was a source of inspiration for him.

"She opened my eyes to how big the world is and taught me the principles of leadership," Joel said. Dr. Ammons was the past president of the International Committee of Sports for the Deaf (ICSD), which was known as Deaflympics.

"Jed and I sent a proposal to ICSD to provide online media for the organization. Dr. Ammons decided to give us a chance, as she believed in both of us," Joel said. "Online media changed everything and brought lots of exposure to the organization. We also started the World Federation of the Deaf's online media. Dr. Ammons taught me that leaders give to others–they can't do everything themselves."

Deep down, Joel had an entrepreneur's heart but he was spreading himself thin among too many endeavors. In the early days of the Internet, Joel did website development and hosting, creating sites for deaf and hard of hearing people as well as providing Internet service. He also produced a newspaper that focused on deaf topics.

One day, Joel and his brother came up with the idea of creating a trade show for businesses that served deaf and hard of hearing people. They envisioned a place where businesses and organizations could connect with deaf customers.

"We wanted to create a trade show with free admission," Joel said. "Sponsors were skeptical about the business model at first."

What happened next was an entrepreneur's dream: DeafNation Expo continued to draw crowd after crowd during the one-day event held in different cities throughout the year. The trade show has expanded to include a DeafNation World Expo held in Las Vegas. The first two World Expos each attracted 42,000 people from all over the world.

"I learned a lesson: when you have a clear focus, your business will grow," Joel said. "Money won't be an issue–you will have steady growth year after year, especially when you centralize your focus."

But remember Joel's dream of working for a major studio? He did something even better. Joel created his own production company within DeafNation, and now he travels all over the world capturing stories of deaf and hard of hearing people living extraordinary lives and sharing them in his show *No Barriers with Joel Barish*.

"I've met different people from all over the world," Joel said. "No one is the same, but there's always one thing we have in common: Deaf pride."

Joel recalled a trip to the Panama Canal, where he stopped to interview employees at a deaf school. The school produced the official flag of Panama, so it was a frequent stop for the media. In the middle of one interview, the deaf employee began to cry.

"What's wrong?" Joel asked.

"This is the first time anyone has interviewed a deaf person at the school," she explained. "The media always interview the staff who can hear."

Joel has traveled to 70 countries and 48 states (North Dakota and Montana are the only two left), and has many more trips planned. His company has produced more than 3,000 videos featuring deaf and hard of hearing people from all walks of life and professions. He doesn't just capture stories, he experiences them firsthand–whether it is harvesting rice, installing auto glass, riding in a fire truck, or climbing a tower.

One year, he invited people to compete for a spot to travel with him to Korea. Fifteen participants won a spot, including a man whose family had begged him to cut off his growing beard for years–he wanted the trip so badly he chopped off his beard during his submission video and ended up being selected to go.

All the interviews Joel has done have inspired him in different ways. Two of his favorites to-date were in Rome, Italy, and Fort Worth, Texas. Joel interviewed Roberto Wirth, owner of Hotel Hassler, in Rome, Italy. Hotel Hassler is a five-star hotel where famous and wealthy people from all over the globe go to stay.

In Fort Worth, Joel talked with airplane mechanics Michael Boland and Robert Bond, who work for American Airlines. Both mechanics have 14 years of experience. What's even more remarkable is that Michael works with just one arm, since his left arm extends just past the elbow. In yet another interview, Joel talked with several Boeing mechanics, including one who has installed more than 1,000 engines.

"Imagine the pilots flying the 777 and 737 planes–they're piloting planes with engines installed by deaf mechanics," Joel said.

Joel works tirelessly to produce his interviews because he knows the stories inspire others to realize their own potential when they see deaf people doing all kinds of amazing things.

"I've never let anything stop me," Joel said. "Deaf kids have so much potential and parents often don't realize how much they can do–they underestimate their children's abilities."

Joel wraps this up with some specific advice for parents: "Don't limit your kid's dreams. If they think they can't do something–push them over their self-imposed limits and they'll accomplish their dreams."

For more of Joel's interviews, visit www.deafnation.com.

CHAPTER 9

SOFIA SEITCHIK: COACHING OTHERS TO SUCCESS

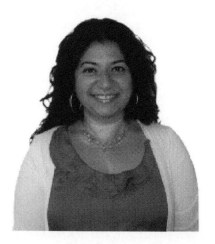

Sofia Seitchik was born in Samarkand, Uzbekistan (which became independent from Russia in 1991), the site of one of the oldest continually inhabited cities in the world and known for its position on the famous Silk Road trade route. Born into a Jewish family of four girls in an Islamic country under a communist regime, Sofia learned from an early age that she stood out.

Her parents learned she was deaf at the age of two and one year later, they enrolled Sofia in a boarding school for deaf children 3,000 miles away from home in St. Petersburg, Russia. From ages 3 to 16, Sofia spent her life at the school from September to

May and saw her family during the summer. Her younger deaf sister, Irina, joined her at the school. The staff and students became their family.

"During communist times, travel was hard," Sofia said. "A one-way plane ticket equaled two months of salary. I have a lot of respect for my mom, she sacrificed so we could have a better education. I know it was hard for her to do this."

During the long years at school, the one thing that kept Sofia going was her dreams.

"I always told myself, 'There is better way of life; I'm here for a reason.' Many times, I wanted to quit life when I was in the institute for too long and not seeing what is out there, but my inner belief and dreams kept me going. I dreamed I could become whatever I wanted to be."

Growing up as a deaf Jewish woman in Russia meant her future was very limited but in her thoughts, Sofia escaped the oppression and dreamed of becoming a teacher. Her parents moved to America in 1989 to give the four girls a better future. Six months before the move, Sofia learned the skill of dressmaking from a private tutor. Three weeks after arriving in New York City, Sofia found a job in a textile factory folding bed sheets. Every day, she walked 30 minutes to the factory in Brooklyn with her Russian-English Dictionary and familiarized herself with her new country and new language. The family soon found the Lexington School for the Deaf and moved to Queens, New York, so the girls could attend the school.

"Everything was such a culture shock for me," Sofia recalled. "When I got into high school, I learned about Deaf culture. I learned about my Jewish heritage and studied for my Bat Mitzvah.

"There was a family culture shock, too. I didn't know my family well after all those years and I was adjusting to being Jewish and within the hearing culture, and spending time 24/7 with my family, who in many ways I barely knew. There were communication challenges as well. I had to learn three languages at once: English,

American Sign Language, and Hebrew. Hebrew was my choice because I was able to be proud being Jewish and able to practice freely in United States and wanted to participate in Bat Mitzvah."

While she was at Lexington, Sofia participated in many after-school activities and programs; one of her favorite activities was acting in mock trials as a lawyer. The Lexington School for the Deaf competed with hearing schools in the mock trials. This activity made Sofia entertain thoughts of becoming an attorney.

She began her college journey at California State University in Northridge with political science as her major, but soon realized becoming a lawyer wasn't for her. She transferred to Gallaudet University to major in communications. After college, she traveled Europe and Asia, worked as a substitute teacher, and then landed a job as the coordinator of community affairs at the Lexington Center for the Deaf.

"That was a fun job," Sofia said. "I hosted many professional events for the deaf professional community and also provided sensitivity training to major corporations, hospitals, fire, and police agencies."

After 9/11, the funding for the job was cut and Sofia transferred as a job coach at Lexington for the next two years and worked as an ASL instructor at Hunter College.

Still, Sofia was itching for more. She loved to travel and had backpacked her way through 30 countries. She left her jobs at Hunter College and Lexington Center for the Deaf, and opened a home-based travel agency. It was a big risk, as she had no background in business or marketing, or working for herself, but she had a lot of common sense and a willingness to learn.

She attended a travel agency business conference that changed her life. There, she met several motivational speakers and learned how they started at the bottom and became successful. She left inspired, but realized she had few people to share it with. While she was in a bookstore searching for motivational books written by deaf people, she realized there was nothing in the bookstore that would specifically motivate deaf and hard of hearing people.

"That was my 'ah-ha' moment," Sofia said. "More and more deaf people were going into their own businesses, but there were no deaf motivational speakers to provide guidance, education, or leadership. As deaf people, we have our challenges just like people who can hear, but there was no one who understood the differences in our challenges–I realized there was a big gap there."

Sofia pursued the path to become a life coach, then later received her business coach certification. She found she enjoyed providing support while helping others identify their dreams and outline a plan to achieve them.

"I found that some people had difficulty dreaming big or they felt they like they couldn't because they are deaf. That's what I see a lot and it breaks my heart," Sofia said. "You can always achieve greater things than you realize. I was fortunate that I had a natural instinct–I didn't believe in limits. I didn't believe in the word 'no.' There's so much out there, so much more than you think–that's what inspired me to become a business transformation coach."

Sofia spends her days teaching others how to achieve their vision and dreams, and provides ongoing support to keep them on track. Her business, Global Deaf Women, works with female entrepreneurs so they can gain confidence, live their passion, achieve their vision, and prosper financially. Many women have benefited from attending Global Deaf Women's Power of Me retreats and her intensive coaching sessions, where they are inspired, find their passion, let go of their past disappointments. and overcome obstacles.

"When I meet someone, they leave a blueprint in me," Sofia said. "I always like to attract positive people–people who are changing the world and people who follow big dreams–they feed me. I wanted to pursue my own big dreams. Today, I work from home, I have a flexible schedule, a beautiful loft I work from every day. Looking back, I'm glad I followed my heart, and not the crowd."

For more information on Sofia's business coaching and Global Deaf Women, visit www.globaldeafwomen.com.

CHAPTER 10

TATE TULLIER: LIFE THROUGH A LENS

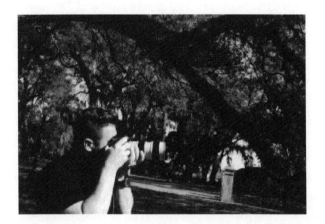

Tate Tullier remembers his first photo shoot very well. As a teen he was fascinated with girls and fashion. One Christmas morning, he dolled up his young cousin with his mom's earrings and an umbrella and proceeded with a fashion shoot. He grabbed another young family friend in her Christmas pajamas and snapped away.

"You can take four pictures, that's it," Tate's mom warned. Digital cameras had not yet arrived on the scene, so Tate had to wait patiently for the film to be developed.

As a deaf teen who grew up with Cued Speech, Tate knew he was different from his guy friends. His friends were into hunting and sports. "I just wanted to take pictures," Tate recalls. "Over the next four years in high school, I kept taking pictures."

Tate was fascinated with fashion and beautiful women. *Vogue* and *People* magazines were his favorites and he begged his mom for a subscription to each. His mom was skeptical–the subscriptions were not cheap and she worried that her son would soon lose interest shortly after subscribing. For Tate, his fascination with fashion and photography grew stronger with every issue he received. He spent hours flipping through the magazines and studying the clothes and photo angles.

"I always had good deaf friends growing up and a great family," Tate said. "My parents tried to get me into sports, but it wasn't me, it wasn't my thing. Magazines, fashion, design, photos–that was me. I was very visual. They let me go with my passion and I found my area of excitement."

Tate met Sarah, the girl who would later become his wife, at a deaf camp in Louisiana. She worked as a lifeguard at the camp pool and, for a short time, they connected over fashion and photography. Tate went off to college, but he found himself daydreaming during his classes. Instead of paying attention to the course material, he was looking around the classroom and contemplating picture angles or studying the architecture around him. He was more fascinated with the people on campus than the stuff he was supposed to be learning. Tate lost a scholarship due to his lack of focus and transferred to a college close to home, where he connected with Sarah again. The couple enrolled at Gallaudet University and continued to grow as a couple. Tate did photo shoots for students at rock-bottom prices and worked at Barnes & Noble on the side. It took him seven and half years to graduate with a degree in visual art and a minor in photography.

Tate's first full-time job took him off-course from his passion: he worked as a recruiter for Gallaudet University and traveled the Midwest. As much as he loved the travel and the people he met on the journey, his heart wasn't the process. Here and there, he began to shoot weddings for friends. A colleague gave him some advice: "Work for yourself."

The path to his own business wasn't an easy one at first. The couple moved to New York and then Louisiana, as Sarah finished up her internship and took a job. Tate continued to do weddings here and there. His business, Tate Tullier Photography, began to take off when Tate posted his photos on Facebook and Twitter. On a whim, Tate took a picture of himself bathing in a tub one night and posted it as "Tub Time with Tate." The tub shots became a signature shot and Tate began to get more and more requests for tub photo shoots.

"Tub shots became my thing–a little risque, but fun," Tate said. "I could be creative with the water, with reflections on the body...it could be interpreted any way you want."

Today, Tate is always on the road doing shoot after shoot and he loves every minute of it.

"Whatever your passion is–just do it," Tate said. "It's so cliche, but just do it. Figure out a way to make it happen and try not to be afraid. Fear is always good. You need to do what you want in your life and don't give up. If you love your job, you don't work a day in your life."

See Tate's photography work at www.tatetullier.com.

CHAPTER 11

THOMAS MCDAVITT: A LOVE FOR ANIMALS

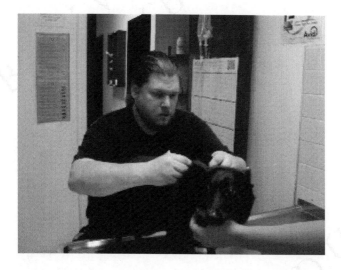

Ever since he was seven years old, Dr. Thomas McDavitt knew he wanted to become a veterinarian. After his pet Labrador Bear died from poisoning, the young man decided that he wanted to be in a profession that saved animals and brought them back to health.

Thomas discovered the path to becoming a veterinarian was filled with obstacles along the way. Deaf since the age of five due to spinal meningitis, he encountered people who tried to discourage him from the profession because of his hearing loss.

"Whenever someone told me I couldn't do something, my response was always a simple, 'Watch me!" he said.

While studying at Kansas State University, Thomas volunteered at the Sedgwick County Zoo, cleaned cages at a teaching hospital, and worked at the immunology lab. A few of his professors expressed concern about the challenges ahead, but Thomas had no doubt he was going to get into veterinary school.

"I was confident in myself and my abilities," Thomas said. Finding a job after college proved to be challenging at first. Thomas found a position at a small clinic in the quad cities area of Illinois and then moved to another clinic in central Illinois. Today, he co-owns the Animal Clinic of Alsip in Illinois, providing services for more than 4,000 clients. Several of his clients are deaf or hard of hearing and Thomas uses sign language to communicate with them. Communicating with his clients can be a challenge at times but he has staff to assist him when needed. The staff also handles phone calls and appointments.

"About the only area that I have difficulty working directly with the animals is when listening to the lungs or heart," Thomas explained. "I use my hands to feel the heartbeat or sometimes I have a staff person listen with a stethoscope to confirm what I feel. If I have any doubt about a diagnosis in those areas, I always refer out."

Laser surgery is his specialty. Few veterinarians in his area have that expertise so clients seek out Thomas for that skill.

When Thomas closes up for the day, he heads home to his wife, daughter, and a house full of pets. He has two dogs, five cats, a ferret, and a lovebird. He didn't plan to end up with so many cats, but clients occasionally abandoned pets at the clinic and Thomas ended up bringing them home. One such abandoned cat is a permanent resident at the clinic. One summer, Thomas found himself caring for one of his elderly dogs after the dog broke its leg. Gangrene set in and with a heavy heart, he had to amputate the dog's leg.

"The dog's doing fine now, hopping around on three legs!" he smiled.

Today, Thomas serves as a role model for deaf and hard-of-hearing children, visiting schools and talking to students about the challenges and rewards of his profession.

"Never let anyone say, 'You can't,' because you can," he said.

CHAPTER 12

KAREN MEYER: REPORTING THE NEWS ON ABC

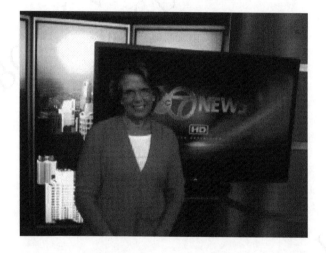

Karen Meyer works at ABC News Channel 7 in Chicago as a reporter. Twice a week, Karen produces, edits, and reports news segments that feature disability topics. Karen is deaf and does not use hearing aids or have a cochlear implant. She speaks and signs during each news segment.

Karen and her younger brother, Gary, were born profoundly deaf. Karen remembers having a "Chatty Cathy" doll at the age of four, and complaining to her mother, "The doll doesn't talk!" She would pull the string, and hear nothing. In reality, the doll was chatting away.

Karen attended Evanston High School, sharing an English class with another deaf classmate. Most of her friends had hearing in the normal range. Finding a job as a teenager was a struggle. For two years, she was unable to convince an employer to see past her hearing loss and take a chance on hiring her. Her mother handled phone calls for both the job interviews and her social life.

"Students today have access to technology which makes communication easier. We didn't have that back then," Karen said. "There are almost no barriers to personal communication today, thanks to technology and current laws. Today, it is cool to be deaf."

Karen tossed aside her hearing aids after wearing a broken hearing aid for a long while and not even realizing the difference.

"I am happy being who I am," Karen said.

College was difficult due to poor communication access in her classes, but Karen made it through by speechreading and borrowing her classmates' notes. After receiving her BA in social work, Karen began exploring different paths in the disability field. She learned sign language while working for North Suburban Special Recreation as a camp counselor. During graduate school, she used interpreters for the first time. She went on to receive her master's degree in urban studies. Karen spearheaded a pilot program for Jewish Family and Community Services and provided counseling to deaf and hard of hearing persons. She eventually started her own consulting firm, focusing on accessibility issues and the Americans with Disabilities Act.

Her path into broadcast journalism was a matter of being in the right place at the right time. After giving a presentation on disability issues at the ABC News Channel 7 station, the manager, Joe Ahern, asked if she would start weekly reports for the station. Karen's first broadcast was mired in controversy when a local radio station grumbled its disapproval about having a reporter with a speech impediment. The ABC station stood by their newest reporter and over the years, Karen has received numerous awards for her reporting.

More than 20 years after that first broadcast, Karen is still reporting 104 stories per year. Karen prepares and edits each segment weeks before it goes on air. When Karen conducts an interview, she relies on lipreading and then has an assistant translate each tape. Early in Karen's career, she used interpreters to assist with communication but as the years rolled by, her co-workers learned to communicate with her. When Karen is on the air, she relies on visual cues from the staff to begin and end her segments. Most of her reporting time averages two to three minutes, which is longer than other segments on the show. She broadcasts the introduction live and adds an ending statement after each tape runs.

"Some of the most memorable broadcasts are those that help people or make a difference in their lives," Karen said.

In one of her broadcasts, Karen featured a 14-year-old teen who stuttered. The young man struggled with the disorder, facing peers who teased him, and using therapy to help him cope. He attended a camp where he learned to rap. In the midst of rapping, he discovered he no longer stuttered.

"I was amazed at this young man," Karen said. "When I first met him, I could feel his pain when he was speaking, and then when he was rapping, I could feel that pain being relieved. I was very proud he found a niche to thrive in a very difficult world."

Karen has interviewed people with all kinds of disabilities, as well as deaf and hard of hearing people. Kathy Buckley, Marlee Matlin, Henry Kisor, and Heather Whitestone have all graced the screen. Ray Charles, Clay Walker, Greg Louganis, and Bob Love are notable others.

For fun, Karen enjoys running and playing tennis. Karen ran her first Chicago Marathon at the age of 44 and has completed five marathons. Today, she plays tennis five days a week and competes in tournaments.

"Anything is possible. You have to make it happen," Karen advised. "Take risks!"

To see some of Karen's broadcasts, visit www.abclocal.go.com/wls (click on "Disability Issues").

CHAPTER 13

MOJO MATHERS: ACTIVE IN GOVERNMENT

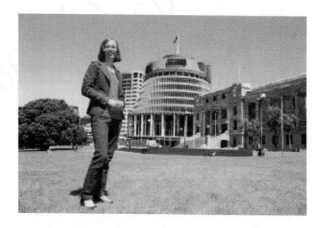

Mojo Mathers didn't intend to go into politics, but when she heard about plans to build a massive dam in a special river near her home in New Zealand, she decided she had to do something about it. She sprang into action and, alongside a group of passionate local people, successfully helped fight the dam and saved the river. Her involvement led to a high local profile and she was invited by the Green Party to run as their candidate for Parliament. Although she was not successful at first, she was elected the the time she ran, becoming New Zealand's first deaf member of Parliament.

Her passion for environmental concerns runs deep.

"I obtained my master's degree in conservation and forestry, with the intention of being a scientist in conservation work," Mojo said. "I'm passionate about protecting the environment and protecting biodiversity."

Mojo was born in England and became profoundly deaf as a result of a lack of oxygen at birth. She didn't take well to hearing aids at first, pulling them out frequently.

"My mother was very aware that with my level of deafness, I wouldn't develop language easily. She knew I would miss out on the small words, so she taught me to read–and at the same time, she taught me to speak," Mojo said. For a short time in primary school, Mojo attended a classroom with other deaf and hard of hearing students. When her family moved, she was placed in a primary school where she was the only deaf student.

"I didn't really have any friends, mainly because the teacher didn't explain to the other children how to interact with a deaf child," Mojo said. "The other children stayed away from me–they did not know how to involve me."

At the age of 11, Mojo went to the Mary Hare School, a boarding school for profoundly deaf children that used an auditory/oral approach in its instruction. Although she was homesick at first and found it hard to adjust to living in a dorm, Mojo found herself enjoying the small classes with other deaf and hard of hearing students.

Three years later, her family moved to New Zealand and she once again found herself in the mainstream, but at a high school with support for deaf students.

"I was lucky: when I arrived at that school, the staff put some students in charge of helping me to integrate and settle in," Mojo said. "I became part of a big peer group who played together–they pulled me in and accepted me. I felt integrated in the school."

Mojo was the dux (valedictorian) of her graduating class.

College was a challenge as Mojo had very little in the way of access or support. She graduated with a degree in mathematics and a master's in conservation and forestry. For five years, she and her husband co-owned a business that offered forestry management services. She became a mom to three children but continued to be involved in community and environmental issues. For years, the family lived in a rural area and Mojo had no contact with other deaf and hard of hearing people.

Then

New Zealand passed a law recognizing New Zealand Sign Language as one of three official languages and teachers began sharing it in classrooms.

"My children came home so excited one day and asked, 'Mommy, do you know sign language? It's so cool!'" Mojo said. "So they started to teach me some basic signs. I was amazed. I wanted to learn more about this, so I started connecting up with the deaf community in Christchurch and found them very welcoming, very willing to share their language. I found it was easy to understand sign language, even though I'm very clumsy in signing myself."

For Mojo, her political career and deaf journey collided at the same time. She became a strong supporter of sign language and accessibility issues.

"I got so far in my political journey and then I came up against barriers–I found if I accepted my identity as a deaf person, that's when I could get past the barriers and be more effective politically," Mojo explained. "I had to claim my identity as a deaf person instead of a hearing-impaired person. I had to be upfront about the accommodations I needed to participate politically–sign language interpreters and note takers."

One of the biggest hurdles she faced when she won her seat as a member of Parliament was the issue of funding for communication access. At first, the government insisted the costs be covered from Mojo's MP budget, but they backed down after a significant public outcry, and now the costs are covered by the wider Parliamentary services budget. Mojo also faced doubt from others who were unsure she could handle the job.

"Many people will make a lot of assumptions about what I can or can't do without checking directly with me," Mojo said. "When I first joined the party and stood as a candidate, many members assumed that I wouldn't be able to cope with the pressures of being an MP because of my hearing loss.

"In fact, I have coped very well indeed, and nothing has come up yet that I haven't had to deal with as part of managing the day to day pressures of being deaf in a hearing world. But there was no way of convincing people that beforehand. I was fortunate to have a strong group of people who valued my participation for my unique perspective as well as policy and analytic skills."

Mojo wrapped it up with a message for others:

One of my favorite quotes is from Ghandi: 'Be the change you want to see in the world.' It's important to have good support—to have people around you who can support you to achieve your goals. It's not always easy to keep believing in yourself. It's also important for deaf people to accept and celebrate the identity that comes with being deaf. There are skills you can get from being deaf that hearing people don't have. For example, you can become good at reading body language of people and interpreting emotions. In terms of jobs, deaf people have learned to concentrate in noisy environments—we can turn off the noise and focus on the work. It's very important to look at deafness in a positive light, not negative. We have skills that others don't have as a result of being deaf.

Chapter 14

ADREAN CLARK: THE PUBLISHING ROUTE

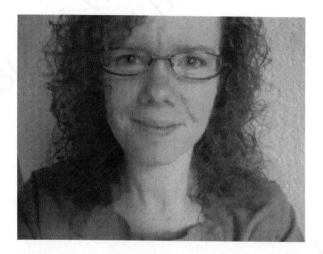

Adrean Clark grew up writing poetry. She also loved to draw and create stories, so comics became a great way to express herself. She never considered turning her skills into a career; the role models in her family were English teachers and librarians, so Adrean considered those paths as a possibility for her future.

Growing up in a mainstream environment was frustrating for Adrean. Attention-deficit/hyperactivity disorder made it difficult for Adrean to sit through the long days with an interpreter in school.

"My personality is very driven and I have a very vivid imagination," Adrean said. "I sat in my seat and fidgeted. I would go on adventures in my mind while watching the interpreter and I would make up stories to cope."

A librarian on Adrean's mother's side of the family had a prediction for her: "You will be a published author."

Writing books seemed like a lot of work–Adrean wasn't interested in the idea at the time, but she found herself intrigued by comics and began to learn how to draw them.

At age 13, Adrean transferred to the Central North Carolina School for the Deaf and learned American Sign Language. She found a connection with her peers by entertaining them with her drawings.

"I would draw cartoons for the other kids. They seemed to really like my art skills, so I kept at it through different schools over the years," Adrean said. "After I graduated from the North Carolina School for the Deaf, I spent some time at Gallaudet and met John Lee Clark, who later became my husband."

After college, Adrean worked as a freelance graphic artist and specialized in comics and cartoons. She enjoyed the freelance work so much she turned it into a career. Then one by one, Adrean began to publish books. She's now on her eighth book.

"With my first book, 'Eight Ways to be Deaf,' I did many comic strips but hadn't put it in a book–so one day I decided 'I'm going to do this!'" Adrean said. "I committed myself five days a week, every day, to finish that book. At the time, I was sick from mold in our home –very sick–and it helped keep my mind off that disease. It took me three months to finish and it was one of the hardest things I ever did, but now I look at it and think, wow–maybe not the drawing I wanted, or the skill level I wanted, but I did it! I set the goal and finished it no matter what."

Adrean a weekly online magazine and from that, she crafted her second book. She found great joy in watching others laugh at her comics. "I love freelancing–I can work for myself or work for other people on my own time," Adrean said. "Because I home-school, I can arrange my schedule around my kids. My husband, John, has Usher syndrome and we use tactile sign, so this work flexibility is valuable for our family–John is a writer, too.

"Sometimes you know what you want and then do it, only to find you don't like it. you have to change direction–you have to find satisfaction– find your challenge and your interests," Adrean said. "It's all right to change the plan as you go along. Every failure is a step toward success."

Find out more about Adrean by visiting www.adreanaline.com.

CHAPTER 15

KATHY BUCKLEY: MOTIVATING THE WORLD

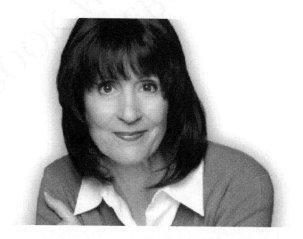

Years ago, Kathy Buckley didn't want to be a comic–she wanted to be an actress. On a dare from some friends, she agreed to perform in a comedy show to raise funds for children with cerebral palsy. For two weeks, she studied other comics and put together a routine. Three comedy rounds later, she claimed fourth place among 80 contestants. From that moment, her career in comedy and public speaking was born. Her comedy brought in numerous awards, including five nominations for Best Female Comedian at the American Comedy Awards.

Life wasn't always a fun ride for Kathy. She started out in life with severe delays with her speech and language development and she was initially placed in a classroom for mentally challenged children. A year later, the professionals had a different diagnosis: Kathy was hard of hearing.

"And they called *me* slow!" she quipped.

Her teen years were rough. Kathy dealt with sexual abuse and suicidal thoughts. One summer day, she lay on the beach soaking up some rays and she didn't hear the rumble of a Jeep heading right toward her. The lifeguard driving the vehicle ran right over her. The rescue squad thought she was dead on the way to the hospital. It took five long years for Kathy to recover from two and half years of intermittent paralysis. Just as life got back on track, she was diagnosed with cancer.

"If you're looking for a safe place in your life, if you're looking for acceptance, if you're looking for love, and looking for respect—you have to look inside first," Kathy explained. "You are the teacher of how you want people to treat you in life. If you play a victim, you will be a victim. If you use your hearing loss as a reason not to succeed, don't blame anybody but yourself."

Kathy's career in motivational speaking began when she took a job with a company that provided Americans with Disabilities Act training. She was given a thick book full of pie charts and complicated terminology.

"I wasn't gonna read a book that thick with pie charts—if it's not apple pie, I know nothing about it," Kathy laughed. "The first time I spoke, I was nervous. My job was to get the corporation interested in hiring people with disabilities. I didn't know what I was talking about—I was so nervous that I ended up letting out a few swear words."

Her boss was not amused. After a short lecture, he decided to give her another chance—this time in front of 200 people. In the middle of the training, Kathy found herself becoming frustrated and nervous again. She looked at the pie chart, looked at the crowd, and slowly put down the pointer.

"I thought to myself, who better knows what it's like to be

rejected by society about something I had no control over," Kathy
said. "Who better knows what it's like to be fired from jobs in the
past because I wasn't comprehending and I wasn't hearing on the
job? Who better knows what it is like when people say I'm not
good enough? That was me–so I decided to share my story."

Kathy shared her struggles to find employment and the barriers she and others faced. She shared success stories as well–stories
of people with disabilities who were going far beyond what any
able-bodied person could do.

"What I was talking about was the human spirit," Kathy said. "I
wanted them to understand you're not hiring people with disabilities–you're hiring their abilities, and that's what the focus should
be on. I burned the pie chart and quit working for the company.
They wanted me to follow the book, but I wanted to follow my
heart. So I became a speaker. My heart belongs to people–my passion is the human spirit."

Kathy's life took another turn when she was performing at a
comedy club one night. The club manager informed her that Tony
Robbins would be arriving at the club that night. Kathy waited
patiently for the well-known motivational speaker to arrive so she
could start her routine.

"I picked on him–I made fun of him being late," Kathy recalled.
"The big motivational speaker doesn't know how to tell time."

After the routine, Kathy met up with Tony in the parking lot
and she shared her admiration for his work helping people. He
invited her to his next conference and asked if she would perform
a comedy routine and allow him to interview her afterward. After
her routine, Tony began asking her questions from the back of the
room.

"I've been up here for a half hour doing deaf jokes and you're
talking to me from the back of the room?" she razzed him.

Kathy began sharing her story–the Jeep accident, the cancer,
the struggles and joys of being deaf–and Tony was speechless when

she was done. He had only known her as a deaf comic; he didn't realize the obstacles she had overcome in life.

"That was over 20 years ago," Kathy said. "I'm one of his Life Mastery speakers–I teach others how to overcome obstacles. Tony and I became like brother and sister. I learned a lot from Tony–I learned to live my passion, to continue to love unconditionally, and to have no expectations of anyone.

"The only person I'm responsible for on this earth is me–and my behavior, and how I want to present myself. I learned that it was okay to be me–I'm Kathy. When I was at Rochester Institute of Technology one time, a student asked me, 'Are you deaf, hard of hearing, or hearing impaired?' I said, 'I'm Kathy. I'm a child of God.'"

One night, Kathy was performing one of her shows and Michelle Christie, a speech therapist who worked with deaf children, approached her. Michelle had created an after-school theater program, No Limits, which was born out of her frustration with the slow progress of speech and language programs for deaf children. Kathy was intrigued with Michelle's program and teamed up with her to work with the kids and raise funds.

"We make it fun for the children to learn," Kathy said. "We have classes that the parents have to go to for 10 weeks in order to keep their kids in this program. Some parents would take four or five buses, four times a week, and we work to get the children caught up to grade level."

Kathy and Michelle want to make sure every child is comfortable being deaf or hard of hearing. It took Kathy 34 long years before she explored and understood all the aspects of being deaf.

"A deaf child often doesn't understand their deafness because it's not visible," Kathy explained. "You can see why a child is in a wheelchair or missing an arm, but you can't see sound–you can't see how much hearing loss a child has. Every child is different–everyone has a different way of learning or comprehending, so we work with the individual needs of that child. I don't care if a child sings, speaks, mimes, sings, or dances–I just believe that every child should have the gift to communicate. Every child should be able to communicate what's in their heart," Kathy said. "There's nothing wrong with being deaf, but there's everything wrong with not being able to communicate. If you play a victim, you will be the victim. If you use your hearing loss as a reason not to succeed, you have no one to blame but yourself."

Kathy spends many of her days traveling from one location to another, speaking to large numbers of people. Some of her events are booked two years in advance. She loves every minute of her life and wouldn't change a thing. Every adversity, every joy, has shaped her into the person she is today.

"You only have one chance at this life, so dream big–live it to the fullest and celebrate each breath you take–in other words, embrace the gift within you," Kathy said.

See Kathy in action at www.kathybuckley.com.

Learn more about the No Limits program at www.nolimitsfordeafchildren.org.

CHAPTER 16

SEAN FORBES AND MARK LEVIN: MAKING MUSIC

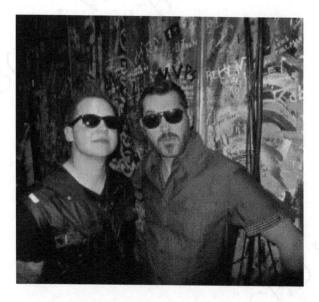

The century-old building was shaking on a Friday night at Columbia College in Chicago. On the stage were three guys: Mark Levin on guitar, Jake Bass on the keyboard, and Sean Forbes belting out a song with his hands flying.

Both Sean and Mark are deaf. Jake is the one with hearing in the normal range–he manages the sound system. The three of them tour the United States together, entertaining audiences in city after city. They're popular, not only because of the energy they exude on the stage, but also because their music is accessible to deaf and hard of hearing audiences. The music is loud and the lyrics are conveyed using American Sign Language.

Sean's parents were both musicians, so he grew up surrounded by music.

Mark's mom gave Mark a guitar for his eighth-grade graduation present and signed him up for private lessons.

"It was always fun for me to play," Mark said. "I didn't see a career at that time–I just wanted to rock! In high school, I took a guitar class with 15 hearing kids and two other deaf kids. That was cool."

Mark played in a friend's band and was hooked. Concerts and music festivals became his escape, and he loved surrounding himself with music. He began to dream of working in the music industry in some way. During a visit with a vocational rehabilitation counselor to discuss his goals for college, Mark shared his vision of graduating with a degree in music, specifically audio engineering.

"That's not a realistic goal," the counselor told him.

However, Mark was determined to hold on to his dream. He couldn't let go of the idea of a career in music, but soon discovered that the engineering aspects of music were not for him. He changed to a focus on art, entertainment and media management. Mark worked two, sometimes three jobs to put himself through college and graduated from Columbia College in 2008 with the coveted music degree.

Mark and Sean's paths crossed through Sean's girlfriend (now wife) who knew Mark from high school. They met at a Blue Man Group concert and forged an instant connection when they found themselves drumming along with the music. Mark joined Sean on stage, and they've been touring together ever since.

"A lot of people out there will say no to you," Mark said. "If you tell me 'no,' no is my fire. I don't like the word no. That word is my motivation–I will find a way to do it. Never say no to yourself.

Roll up your sleeves, do the hard work, pour your blood, sweat, and tears into it and will pay off–it will be worth it."

Everywhere they go, the two of them have inspired people to live their dreams. When they're on stage, they're fueled by the energy from the crowd and the sparkle they see in the eyes of their audiences.

"One situation popped up when I was in New York City, one kid came up to me and said,'I've been bullied– d o you have any advice?' I told him first of all, you have to embrace who you are," Sean said. "I had a similar situation when I was a teen. For most of my life, I hated being deaf. I couldn't connect with my hearing friends or my deaf friends."

When he was 16, Sean had an epiphany that changed everything for him. He woke up one morning with a realization: he was going to be deaf the rest of his life.

"Once I accepted that, life became a lot easier. People would make fun of me, but I would brush it off. 'Yeah, I'm deaf and so what'–once they realized they couldn't get to me, the bullying and teasing stopped," Sean said. "It's all about how you handle it."

Sean advised the young kid to do the same–to be proud of himself and brush off the bullies.

"Treat people how you want to be treated," Sean said. "If you make fun of people, expect negative to come back to you–be positive."

Sean shared more:

I feel like my mission in life is to change people. The older I become, the more I realize I really want to make a difference in people's lives by sharing my background and my history. I want to be one of those people who inspire and change people's perspective–I want to open doors.

Hearing people see what I do with music–in some cases, they've never seen a deaf person before and it changes their perspective of what deaf people can do. The Deaf community is supportive of what I do, and the hearing community is starting to be more open. They want to learn our language. There's more ways for the two communities to connect than before–now we have social media, which helps get to know more about each other through that.

The more I go out, the more I perform, the more I share my story, the more I become open to other possibilities. I love doing what I do–that's what makes my music career worthwhile. When I first started, I wanted to be famous and be on MTV, but I took a different path and I realize my life was in my hands and I could create it any way I wanted to.

My proudest moment is setting up D-PAN and the music video camps we host. When I do the camp and see the kids who showed up, at first, they have no real soul but when they leave, they are smiling and they've discovered something about themselves– that's what makes everything worthwhile. I love how everything is overlapping in my life and how my music is making an impact on people.

The message of 'Don't let anything hold you back' speaks to everyone. My songs are my life stories–they tell the story of overcoming obstacles and still achieving dreams. More and more, I'm writing songs about real-life situations. I come from a divorced family. My stepmother supported me all the way–she taught me how to speak and developed language for me. I try to inspire kids and families through my music by telling parents it's okay to advocate for your child and get the best possible education. With my music, I share stories within stories. The more I do this type of thing, the more I realize that it's really awesome. I never looked up to other musicians who are just about partying and having fun; it's about having fun and being silly, but mixing that with positive messages instead of negative ones.

Today, the guys are living their dream life, traveling around the country and playing music to their hearts' content. The rest of the time, they're working on new songs and belting out tunes in their studio back home in Michigan. And they're also doing something else: everywhere they go, they inspire young deaf and hard of hearing people to listen within… and follow their dreams.

"I've gotten to where I am today because of hard work and dedication. If you have a dream, only YOU can achieve it," Sean said. "Carve your own path, don't be like anyone else."

Keep up with the tour at www.deafandloud.com.

CHAPTER 17

KEVIN DESILVA: ADVENTUROUS ENTREPRENEUR

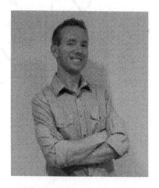

Kevin DeSilva still remembers his first taste of being teased while growing up. It happened on the basketball court in the park while playing with his brother.

"Opposing players would call me names and explode in laughter when I didn't turn my head around to hear what they said," Kevin recalled. Kevin attended the Phoenix Day School for the Deaf and entered Gallaudet University when he was 17. Two years later, he saw a flier from Booz Allen Hamilton, a Fortune 500 company, advertising for summer interns. He went to the career center to apply, but the counselor ended up canceling his interview appointment with the company, stating his resume was too poorly written to submit it.

"She was right," Kevin said. "I didn't know how to write a

resume, so I wasn't upset, but the counselor didn't know my heart. I drove to Booz Allen Hamilton's sprawling campus in Virginia and found my way to HR department." Kevin wrangled an interview and was offered the position.

"Let me tell you, the adviser's face looked as white as a ghost when the recruiter informed her I was offered the position," he chuckled. Kevin enjoyed his experience with the company, but discovered he was bored after a few weeks.

"It was difficult to build rapport with managers due to my deafness," Kevin said. "I'm a confident person and friendly, but still there was something missing. It's a *lot of hard work* to climb the ladder in corporate America."

Three years later, Kevin flew to Sweden as a foreign exchange student. One night, a friend suggested he attend a business meeting in the next town.

"My friend couldn't make it, but my gut said 'you must go,' so I went," Kevin said. He walked into a conference room filled with about 70 people and sat down. Everyone was dressed in professional attire. There was no sign language interpreter and the presenters spoke Swedish, so Kevin didn't understand a word. It was a cold night, so he figured he would sit a bit longer and thaw out before heading back out.

Then a woman in a wheelchair was pushed up the stage. She was young, in her 30s, and sported a happy look on her face. Suddenly everyone applauded and stood up, giving her a long standing ovation. Kevin turned to a man sitting next to him and asked him what was going on. The man told him the woman was very successful in the network marketing business. Kevin didn't pursue network marketing at the time, but he filed away the experience in his mind.

Back in the United States, Kevin began reading books by successful people to try and understand the process of becoming successful. When Kevin picked up the book, *Rich Dad, Poor Dad*, he had no idea his life was about to go down an entirely new path.

"I love stories," Kevin said. "The book is based on different stories from the first to the last page–all stories–no preaching, 'You must do this or you must do that.' That kind of approach is the best way of getting through to people."

The book inspired Kevin to buy his first property and rent it out. He went on to buy two more properties and added more renters.

Kevin continued to learn by reading more and more books and studying successful people. Opportunities for network marketing began to pop up here and there. He remembered the woman in a wheelchair from Sweden and how successful she became in her network marketing business. Kevin dove into network marketing and began building a vitamin business one person at a time. His business grew little by little. After a while, he began to realize he was playing life too safe.

"I didn't realize I was capable of doing more–and doing bigger things," Kevin said. "If something looked very scary, I used to tell myself, 'That's not for me, that's for someone else.' I would give up that opportunity for other people to take. Thanks to reading books on self-development and meeting successful people, I began to realize when you plant seeds, you will eventually reap what you harvest."

After reading Jerry Colangelo's book, *How You Play the Game*, Kevin got in touch with the Phoenix Suns and Diamondback owner and arranged to meet with him to share an idea for reaching out to people with disabilities.

"He was a little nervous meeting me, it really showed me that he is a human being, I'm a human being–we are equal on the playing field. I came away from the meeting realizing, wow, I can do much more," Kevin said.

Kevin also met with Larry Winget, author of *Shut Up, Stop Whining and Get a Life*, and Sharon Lechter, co-author of *Rich Dad, Poor Dad*, the book that launched him into entrepreneurship.

"What I've learned from running my network marketing business is the industry is about empowerment," Kevin said. "This kind of business competition is more encouraging and nurturing–they want everyone to succeed. People with disabilities have a shot at this kind of industry. Everything to run your business is supplied to you.

"Joining this kind of industry showed me how much I didn't know–before that, I thought I knew a lot. I read a lot of books, but there were many things I didn't know–how to communicate with people, how to build relationships, how to lead a training session–I had to learn to improve my leadership role. I learned leadership skills from network marketing."

Kevin took a six-day coaching program with Simon Chan, one of the top distributors in his network marketing company. Simon grew up in New York City, attended Coleman University, and became a NBA basketball player. Simon worked his way to the top in the network marketing company, selling 25 million products, and he averages 600 to 700 new distributors every week.

"I spent a lot of money to gain experience, but it was worth it," Kevin explained. "I observed how Simon built his business and prioritized his life, putting family first. I was inspired by him."

Kevin has big goals to reach the top in his business and he's passionate about helping others do the same.

"Success means you find the right balance," Kevin said. "You get up in the morning, do some meditation, read books, make breakfast with the family, and find time for work, find time for your body, and time for your soul. My goal is to master that balance–people who master that are very successful people."

Connect with Kevin by visiting his website at www.deafentrepreneur.com.

CHAPTER 18

ANN MEEHAN: A THRIVING REALTOR BUSINESS

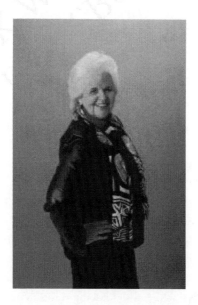

Ann Meehan found herself walking through the model homes every time a new housing development popped up. She was fascinated with everything: the decor, the floor plans, and the prices.

When it came time to sell her own house to move closer to a school for her daughters, Ann became frustrated with the realtor she worked with.

"Because I'm deaf, we wrote back and forth, but I felt like I was missing a lot of information about the selling process," Ann said. "I knew there was more to it than what the realtor was sharing with me."

Ann started calling real estate agencies and located a realtor who had some sign skills. This time, the home-buying experience was a pleasant one. In the process of looking at homes, Ann discovered she was giving her realtor more ideas than what she was getting in return.

"Why don't you become a realtor?" her realtor asked.

At the time, Ann was in business school and had plans to set up a tea shop in town. So at first, she put her networking skills (she owns two network marketing businesses) to work and began by referring clients to her realtor. Little by little, she became drawn to the real estate business and obtained her license.

"I feel like the real estate career fell into my lap," Ann said. "I enjoy people and I enjoy looking at homes. Being a realtor is like a counselor–I have to deal with people's emotions involved."

Through word-of-mouth and referrals, Ann's business began to grow. Eleven years later, The Signing Group is well known in the Frederick, Maryland, area and serves three states. Two of Ann's daughters (one who is also deaf) joined the business, and Ann has plans to add more realtors to handle the growing demand for home sales.

"We use text, email, and videophones to negotiate deals and communicate with our customers and other realtors," Ann said.

Ann still has the dream of opening a tea shop someday, but that will have to wait a while. She's having too much fun with her current businesses.

CHAPTER 19

CJ JONES: A LIFE OF LAUGHTER

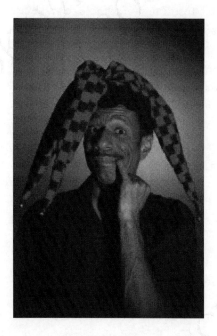

"I was born to be a comedian," CJ Jones said. "When I was five, I watched my brother tap dancing on a Mississippi riverboat and everyone was laughing. I was fascinated. I wanted the same thing–I wanted to make people laugh."

At that time, CJ had hearing in the normal range, along with his two sisters and four brothers. Meningitis struck at the age of seven and CJ became deaf. His deaf parents rejoiced.

During high school, Richard Reed, an English teacher, took CJ
under his wing and taught CJ to love the written word. CJ became
a reporter for the school newspaper and began writing stories and
poems.

"Before I knew it, I was involved with the Literary Society
and that opened up a lot of possibilities for me," CJ said. "Every
Wednesday night, I found myself on stage, exploring ways to play
with English and sign language. I also discovered my leadership
skills at an early age."

CJ took off for New York to study computer programming
at the Rochester Institute of Technology and performed with the
National Theatre of the Deaf. In college, one of his mentors, Bob
Panera, was instrumental in teaching him how to take English
words and convey them beautifully in sign language.

"Bob was a wonderful storyteller," CJ said. "People couldn't
move out of their seats when he performed. I watched him and
learned from him–I wanted to entertain people in the same way."

After CJ graduated from the National Technical Institute for
the Deaf, he took a job in the social service field. He worked as
a director of employment development, placing deaf and hard of
hearing people in various jobs. He found the job challenging, but
discovered he loved motivating and uplifting the clients he worked
with. Happy clients were easier to place in jobs. He received awards
for his motivational speaking and his work.

CJ developed a summer sign language program to bridge the
connections between the corporate world and his clients. The program became immensely popular, but it created a conflict with his
position at work and CJ found himself becoming more and more
frustrated with the confines of his job. Company morale was low
and CJ struggled to stay positive from day to day. Then one day, he
arrived at work to learn the news that he was fired.

"I rolled up my sleeves and fought to get my job back," CJ said.
"Months went by, the case was dropped and I got my job back with
back pay."

One night, he stood on stage performing a comedy routine and all evening, he floated on a natural high from his audience's smiles and laughter. When he arrived at work the next day, his heart sank to his knees. He knew he couldn't go on–the job was sucking his soul dry. CJ submitted his resignation just a month after returning to his job.

"That performance in the community–that's where I belonged. I was happy and my energy was clean and pure. I realized, *that's my destiny!*" CJ said.

CJ has been living his dream for more than 35 years, traveling all over the world to spread laughter and smiles.

"If I was still working a regular job, I would not be happy," CJ said. "I believe that's why I got sidetracked with that job–I lost myself. It was the wrong spot. When I quit–I was either going to make it or not– it was a gamble, but I felt, 'I must do it.' I'm glad I listened to my inner self."

Life has been a whirlwind for CJ. He was cast as Orin in *Children of a Lesser God* and toured the United States and Canada for two years. The cast received a group Tony award for their performances.

CJ also appeared on NBC's *Frasier*, ABC Family's *Lincoln Heights*, the PBS television shows *Sesame Street,* and *Rainbow's End,* and was the host of *Happy Hands Kids Klub*. He has even done voice-over roles, voicing a Deaf Indian (played by a hearing actor) in a movie called *PathFinder* from 20th Century Fox. CJ is one of four Deaf performers showcased in the 2010 documentary *See What I'm Saying* and he also appeared in the documentary *Through Deaf Eyes* on PBS.

He produced the International Sign Language Theater Festival, two children's plays at Deaf West Theater, and currently working on "Once Upon a Sign" children's classics in ASL videos for Dawn Sign Press. When he's not on the road, he's deeply involved in producing videos for his business, Sign World TV, with the dream of turning it into a 24/7 channel on the Internet and television.

"To function in this world, it has nothing to do with being hearing or deaf: it has to do with your humanity," CJ explained. "You contribute to this earth. So many feel they are limited in their contribution—we have so much to contribute, why limit that? Years ago, I made a choice as to what I wanted to do and be—it is my determination as to what creates me. I'm proud I created myself well. My gift, and why I'm here on earth in the first place, that's something I've learned and discovered to understand; my passion, and what I do to entertain and inspire others, that's a gift."

Learn more about CJ by visiting www.cjjoneslive.com.

CHAPTER 20

TINA CHILDRESS: THE AUDIOLOGIST WHO WENT DEAF

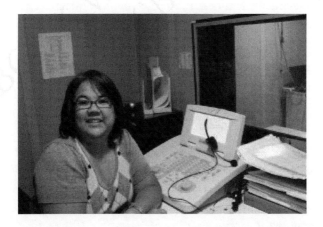

Tina Childress remembers the moment she discovered her own progressive hearing loss. She was working as an audiologist in a school and assisting another audiologist, testing a student. The sounds were coming through the speakers and she noticed the student responding to them, but she couldn't hear them. After the student left, she asked her colleague to do a hearing test and the results showed a mild-to-moderate hearing loss.

Tina's hearing continued to fluctuate and she was eventually diagnosed with autoimmune inner ear disease, a condition that shows up in less than 1 percent of all hearing loss diagnoses. A few months after being diagnosed, she became deaf and could no longer use the telephone. Despite being in a signing environment on the job, she struggled with the speech perception testing and relied on others to listen in. She also found it difficult to conduct listening tests with her students' hearing aids. Over time, she opted for bilateral cochlear implants and was able to use the phone again.

"My epiphany was that I could take this experience and use it to help others with my dual perspective as an audiologist and late-deafened adult," Tina said. "Not only are people feeling overwhelmed as they or their loved ones are going through the grieving process of hearing loss, but they're also inundated with so much jargon and information. I try to take a holistic approach to talking with individuals, families, and professionals to help them realize we need to look at the whole person–audiologically and emotionally–not just fix their ears."

Tina shared more:

One day a group of kids from one of the co-ops I serve came in for their annual hearing test. I was sitting at a table talking to one of the students who was in high school and used hearing aids. This student had known me since the beginning of my career (when I had normal hearing), when I had hearing aids and at the time of this hearing test, I had my cochlear implants. I casually brushed my hair back because it was getting in my eyes and noticed that the student was staring at me wide-eyed and seemingly incredulous. I asked him, 'What's wrong?'

He replied, 'You have cochlear implants!'

I said, 'Yes, I got this one a few years ago and got this one more recently. It really has helped me so much to hear better. Do you remember how deaf I was when I had hearing aids?'

His teary response was, 'Yeah, you really understand what we're going through, don't you?'

It was that a-ha! moment when he realized that I truly could empathize with his communication struggles. I think back to that moment often, especially when I do presentations and training because it really adds another dimension to what I'm trying to teach the audience.

Tina grew up with a love of music and even after becoming deaf, she continued to immerse herself in music, especially with musicals. She successfully advocated for captioned and interpreted access for various venues and continues to promote this wherever she goes.

"I love that I am able to share this love for music with my children and husband, and am known in the deaf or hard of hearing community as 'that musical theater addict,'" Tina laughed. "Yes, I have seen the musical *Wicked* *cough* more than a dozen times and other musicals multiple times as well. I think my greatest joy is when I introduce someone, hearing, deaf, or hard of hearing, to musical theater for the first time and they realize that they can enjoy it whether they can hear or not."

It's also pretty safe to say that Tina is an app addict as well. Her computer, iPad, and mobile phone might as well be attached to her hip. She's a popular expert when it comes to apps that are deaf- or hard of hearing-friendly and she maintains a resource site titled Getting From Hear to There.

"Rather by accident, I started collecting links to apps that can be used by individuals with hearing loss and this list has been shared worldwide," Tina said. "I am very proud of it. I also enjoy helping people understand how assistive technology can help them reach their communication potential. For some, it means assistive listening devices and for others, it's realizing how to leverage technologies like mobile devices and iPads to bring spoken language into a visual form (ASL or text)."

Tina lives by one of her favorite quotes by Goethe: "Whatever you can do or dream you can, begin it. Boldness has genius, power and magic in it."

Visit Tina's blog, Getting from There to Hear, at tinachildress.wordpress.com.

CHAPTER 21

RONNIE CUARTERO: BIKING
SOLO ACROSS AMERICA

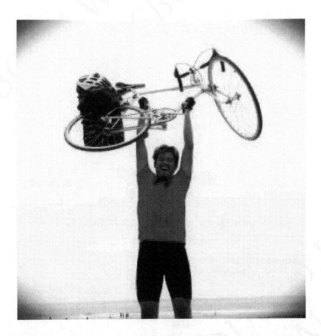

In the summer of 2012, Ronnie Cuartero, a computer major at the Rochester Institute of Technology, and several deaf friends planned to bike from New York to California together. As the trip drew near, his buddies began to back out one by one.

Not Ronnie.

He was determined to ride across America, but he would have

to do it solo. The trip was a challenging one, he admitted. Just 30 minutes into the start of the trip, he wanted to give up. He was already tired and worn out; he couldn't imagine how he was possibly going to face the thousands and thousands of miles ahead of him. For days and days, he churned the pedals over and over, averaging 80 to 100 miles per day. Along the way, strangers reached out, offering him drinks and food. When his bike broke down along a field in Ohio, a friendly farmer delivered him to town and the local bike shop put his 1970s bike back together again.

Ronnie couldn't whittle away the time listening to music or the radio, so he immersed himself in the landscape as each mile passed by. The endless miles brought forth a deep test of patience, determination, and will. Every passing mile looked the same as the next one.

Ronnie had no sponsors, no publicity, and wasn't biking for a noble or charitable cause. So what made him take on such an ambitious solo endeavor?

"I did it for *me*," he said. "I wanted to see America up close. This is something I wanted to be able to look back on years later and say, 'I did it!'"

Here and there, Ronnie stayed with friends for the night or checked into a hotel. In Indiana, he was caught in a torrential rainstorm in the middle of nowhere. Cars whipped by him, splashing him continuously. Ronnie took refuge in a nearby church to wait for the rain to subside. Everything was soaking wet, so he knocked on a nearby door and the homeowners were kind enough to dry his clothes and give him Ziploc bags to seal them in.

"People on the trip were more than friendly–offering discounts at restaurants or free food and drinks," Ronnie said. Ronnie conversed with everyone by writing back and forth using paper and pen. He met some diverse folks along the way, including some from the Amish community.

"I didn't know anything about the Amish way of life when I

started this trip," he said. "I was fascinated to learn they live without electricity and the many things that we take for granted."

By the time he arrived in the Chicago area for a break, he had biked more than 600 miles and still faced 2,400 more. He had just two shirts, two bike shorts, and a pair of pajamas in his bike pack–and he inadvertently left the pajamas behind at his last stop.

"I've learned I can do without many of the things we think are necessary in life," Ronnie said. "We are so used to being comfortable. This trip taught me to survive with very little."

Near the Mississippi River on the way to Iowa, Ronnie stopped at a gas station to rest a bit and grab a drink. A man decked out in riding gear cruised up on a bike and scouted out the bags packed on Ronnie's bike.

"Hi, I'm Bruce. Are you on a bike trip?" he asked. Ronnie shared his bike plans with him.

"I took a similar long-range biking trip with my wife," Bruce said. "We rode from Texas down to Columbia."

The two of them wrote back and forth a bit and then he invited Ronnie to his house. It was a bit hard to converse as they rode, but Bruce did his best with gestures. Ronnie found he enjoyed the company on the ride. When they arrived at the house, he led Ronnie to his garage, which was filled with many different bikes. Bruce and his wife loved to ride and he shared stories of their trips. They wrote back and forth for a half hour.

"I welcomed the break and the company on the ride," Ronnie said. "He inspired me the rest of the trip–just knowing that someone else out there had accomplished their dreams. After that, I never once thought of giving up."

Despite the new enthusiasm, Ronnie found Iowa a challenge. He faced temperatures over 100 degrees, with 80 percent humidity and frequent hills. To top it off, he became sick and had to pull over several times to empty his stomach. He had no strength left and decided to wave for help. Car after car zipped by him, and no one stopped for several hours. Ronnie decided to do something he had never done before: he prayed.

A few minutes later, a car pulled over and a woman asked if he needed help. She offered him a ride to the nearest gas station and Ronnie gratefully accepted.

"Before she dropped me off, I just had to ask her–what made her stop to help me?" Ronnie said. "The woman explained that she doesn't usually stop to help people on the road, but when she saw me, she felt God told her to stop and help. I will never forget that. Before this trip, my faith was not strong. I did a lot of thinking about God after that."

Although he was still weak, he hit the road again. Ronnie didn't have much of a choice at that point; he had to keep powering on through the endless miles. Despite fires were burning in Colorado and a slight diversion, Ronnie found it easier to bike through the mountain states. The downhill coasting carried him far.

As he neared the end of his trip, Ronnie had to dig deep down through the exhaustion to push himself forward with every mile.

"I wanted the end to hurry up and get here," Ronnie said. "I had suffered so much and I had no energy left. But the closer I came to the end, the more energized I became, especially when I saw my friends and family waiting for me."

A wave of emotion enveloped him when he got off the bike. Ronnie had accomplished the incredible feat of biking from New York to California completely by himself. It was at that moment he realized he could accomplish anything he set his mind to.

"You have to suffer to reach your goals and dreams," Ronnie said. "Not many are willing to do what I did, but I got a great sense of accomplishment from doing it.

"Smiling is the easiest way to make life easy."

CHAPTER 22

JAY BLUMENFELD: A BUSINESS IN GREETING CARDS

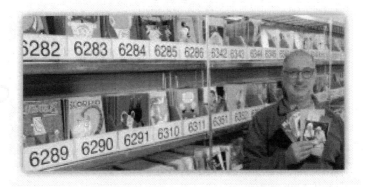

Jay Blumenfeld is the owner of Smart Alex, a business that specializes in alternative greeting cards with off-color humor you'd never find at Hallmark.

Jay never intended to start a greeting card business. As a teen, he was fascinated by photography and thought he might follow in his father's footsteps as a professional photographer.

"My father owned a photo lab and worked as a photographer, but ironically, I taught myself most of my photography skills. I practiced on my own," Jay said. "In order to experiment with lighting and backgrounds, I recruited my family members and friends as models."

Jay won many awards for his photography, including a contest for *Seventeen* magazine.

One month before he was due to graduate with his AAS degree, Jay encountered a bully who threatened him to the point where he didn't want to go anywhere on campus. After he received his degree, Jay was too distraught to return to the same college for his bachelor's degree. Instead, he began working for his father as a photographer.

After two years, Jay was looking for a fresh start, so he moved to Chicago. Jay's photography skills led him to put together a book featuring highly fashionable cross-dressers. Day after day, he scoured the literary agents and publishing houses in New York to find a publisher willing to take on the book. One by one, publishers made similar comments to Jay: "The photographs in your book would make an excellent greeting card for the alternative market."

Jay pondered the idea and thought it would be a great way to get the attention of publishers and agents–and perhaps lead to the opportunity to publish his book. Jay consulted with a printer and estimated he needed $5,000 to start printing greeting cards. He went to his father and asked to borrow money, but his father wasn't confident in his business idea. He arranged for financing from a bank and printed 10 different cards. To his surprise, they all sold out quickly. He borrowed more money, and his business began to grow. From there, Smart Alex was born.

"I had no business training–I learned everything from scratch," Jay said. "When I first met the guy who became my accountant, he was filled with doubts after learning that I had no background in business. He didn't think I would make it through the first year, because 80 percent of new businesses fail after the first year. But here I am, 33 years later and still going strong!"

Smart Alex has sold more than 19 million cards in some major department and retail stores. One of his cards even made it on the Letterman show.

"I don't travel the world, I don't own a fancy house, but what thrills me the most is knowing that 19 million people have bought my cards and smiled and laughed," Jay said.

Jay encourages other deaf and hard of hearing people to go into business, but he cautions them to go into it for the right reasons.

"You have to have a passion and a plan for your business and not just in it to make money," he said. "Deaf people today have it so much easier than years ago. When I started my business, I had to depend on other people to make phone calls for me or I had to drive to offices to network–there were a lot of barriers back then. Today, we have email access and if you need an answer, there's always Google!

"The most important lesson is that you have to believe in yourself," Jay continued. "People will criticize you–listen to them, maybe change a bit, but still believe in yourself. Never let people push you down. I've always listened to my intuition. If I listened to my critics years ago, I wouldn't be as successful as I am today."

Check out Jay's cards at www.smartalexinc.com.

CHAPTER 23

HOWARD ROSENBLUM: A CAREER IN JUSTICE

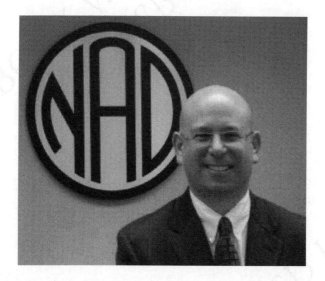

One evening, Howard Rosenblum's mother tried hard to convince her 12-year-old son to attend an event at their synagogue but he stubbornly insisted on staying home. There was no way he was going to give up an evening parked in front of the TV to go and watch some deaf guy give a presentation.

A short time after his mother left, she returned with his school classmate, Marlee Matlin, in tow.

"You need to come back with us to keep Marlee company," she

said. Howard grudgingly joined them. Little did he know, it was a night that would change his life.

Howard sat in amazement and watched Lowell Myers narrate his life as a deaf attorney. With a background in law and finance, he worked for Sears Insurance Company in a Chicago office housed in the Sears (now Willis) Tower. On the side, he handled legal situations for many deaf and hard of hearing clients.

During Lowell's presentation, Howard had an "ah-ha!" moment: Deaf people can sue hearing people!

"Thank goodness my mom forced me to go," Howard said. "My mom *always* told me that I could be a doctor or a lawyer, but watching Lowell–who was living a real life story–I felt like I could relate.

"That was an amazing concept for me," Howard continued. "I did see deaf adults at the synagogue, but in my mind, hearing people had all the power. Watching Lowell present woke me up–after that, I saw more and more deaf people in leadership roles."

Howard became deaf at the age of two due to spinal meningitis and, at first, his parents struggled to adapt.

"For my parents, it was a big surprise to them–they had never met a deaf person before. My mother was a teacher; she had to figure out what was the best thing for me and looked at the options. What she discovered was, there are no 'right' answers. My whole family learned to sign and my mom made sure I learned English well. My mom, however, has sign dyslexia," Howard grinned.

During middle school, Howard shared the story of meeting Lowell Myers with someone at his school and announced he wanted to become a lawyer as well.

"The staff person never said 'You can't,' but her expression said it all," Howard recalled. "I looked at the staff person and thought, 'You think I can't?' It made me determined to prove them wrong. Maybe that's what I needed, but what if it happened to another kid and it crushed their self-esteem? Since that time, my message to all parents and teachers has been this: Raise your expectations, don't lower them."

After Howard graduated from high school, he knew without a doubt that a career in law was for him but decided to get his undergraduate degree in engineering before going to law school. After law school, Howard passed the bar exam and with the engineering degree and law license, he planned to focus on intellectual property law. He applied to 20 different firms, but received no call backs or offers. Disability and special education law practices wanted him, so Howard decided to shift his focus for a short time and try that field. He took a job with a private law firm.

"I knew discrimination and I knew what it was like not to be able to practice law in my choice of the field, so I wanted to address the overall discrimination," Howard said. "I decided to try disability law for a short time, but the more I worked in it, the more I liked it."

After working at a private firm for ten years, Howard became a staff attorney at Equip for Equality.

When Howard received his law license, Lowell Myers had retired and deaf and hard of hearing people flocked to Howard for advice and legal assistance. Howard struggled to find specialized lawyers to handle their cases, but found resistance in convincing those lawyers to take on deaf clients. He asked a former law school classmate to work with a deaf client who needed a divorce. The attorney was hesitant at first.

"I asked him to take the case, but I made him a deal," Howard explained. "If it went well and he liked it, I would refer every divorce case involving a deaf or hard of hearing person to him, and he would be able to build a niche. If he didn't, I wouldn't bother him again."

As it turned out, the case went well and so did many more after that. The classmate asked Howard to continue to give him more cases.

"I gave him as many as I could, but I couldn't force deaf people to get a divorce," Howard chuckled.

Due to the growing demand for accessible legal services for deaf clients, Howard set up a nonprofit organization, the Midwest Center for Law and the Deaf and hired a person to staff the referrals.

Along the way, Howard never forgot how Lowell Myers' presentation charted a course in his life. He wanted to do the same for deaf and hard of hearing children, so he set up presentations with local schools and began to share his story. He was startled when a deaf student expressed doubt that a deaf person could be a lawyer and asked him, "Are you hearing?"

Howard realized he had a mission: he wanted to give deaf and hard of hearing children the same vision and hope for the future that he'd experienced with Lowell. The mission grew into the Adult Role Models in Education for the Deaf program (ARMED) at the Chicago Hearing Society. Howard, in turn, has inspired many others to become lawyers. Today, there are more than 300 deaf and hard of hearing lawyers.

"I want deaf kids to know they can achieve whatever they want–being deaf or hard of hearing should not stop anyone. Society believes in limitations, but that's true of all people–people of different races, gender, religions, etc.," Howard said. "We have to dispel those misguided beliefs and show them what we can do. Parents need to expect the same for all their children, whether deaf or hearing."

Today, Howard is the CEO of the National Association of the Deaf, a position in which he feels he can make a greater impact for deaf and hard of hearing people on a larger scale. The NAD has made great strides in the disability rights arena, working on several different issues at once.

"I enjoyed my 19 years as an attorney in Chicago," Howard said. "I sued many places for disability access–a lot of those places were hospitals, but I often felt like a mouse on a never-ending wheel. In many cases, there would be changes for the better and places would become accessible to deaf and hard of hearing people, but then due to staff turnover, those places would go back to the same discriminatory practices. At the National Association of the Deaf, I can go beyond the legal aspects and use political channels to change the system."

The NAD was also instrumental in changing federal regulation of the trucking industry for deaf and hard of hearing drivers. As a result, 40 drivers obtained their CDL license to drive trucks.

"This is my passion–my work has been driven by what I see with all the challenges and barriers that deaf and hard of hearing people face," Howard said. "My work inspires me to make things change–which benefits so many people–myself included. I have been fortunate to visit other countries–and I see deaf and hard of hearing people in those countries face more significant barriers than what we face in the United States. Many of them are where we were 50 years ago.

"Seeing such barriers in other countries make me appreciate what we have already achieved, but we nevertheless have a long way to go before we achieve true equality. At the NAD, we have lots of goals and plans ahead of us. Life has so many challenges and we have to do what we can to create the change that we want to see, within limits, of course. There's a saying, and I'm paraphrasing it, but it goes like this: 'People plan, God laughs.'"

Find out how you can get involved by visiting www.nad.org.

TO WRAP UP

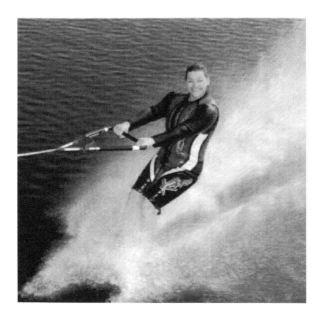

SHARING MY STORY

There's just one more story to share: mine.

As far as I can tell, I was born with hearing in the normal range. As a youngster, I remember crawling into bed and listening to my dad tell me stories about Scamp and Tiny, two little dogs who went on adventures all over town. Then one day, I crawled into bed and could no longer understand him well. I had become sick with a high fever and this had destroyed some of the hair cells in my cochleas. Like a piano with broken keys, I could no longer under-

stand some words without visual cues. I stopped using the telephone and began to pick up the skill of lipreading.

I didn't get my first hearing aid until I was nine. How I hated
that thing. The mechanical sounds produced by the plastic piece
of wired technology simply jarred my brain. The words coming
through still didn't make much sense–they were just louder. I liken
this experience to taking all the consonants out of a sentence.

Go ahead and try it–you'll soon find that you can't read a sentence with just vowels. However, take the vowels out of a sentence
and you can easily figure out what is being said. This is why some
folks have such good use of residual hearing than others–some of
us are getting consonants and able to fill in the blanks and some of
us are getting only vowels and understanding nothing.

I hardly ever wore the hearing aid. As soon as I arrived home
from school, I tossed it on a shelf. During the summer, it gathered
dust. I struggled to understand what was being said in school and
with groups–the struggle just became a way of life. I learned to
develop elaborate systems to fit in and function as "normally" as
possible. During one class, the teacher had each of us take turns
reading a paragraph out of a textbook. I counted the number of
students ahead of me and calculated which paragraph would be
mine to read. I had to listen carefully, as sometimes a student
would be prompted to read two short paragraphs. Never mind the
amount of sweat that poured out just to appear like everyone else;
when it was my turn, I read on cue.

I tried so hard to fit in that I became the queen of social bluff-
ing. A thoughtful nod, a smile and a laugh were the tools I used to
blend in with crowds and have a great, yet lonely, time.

In high school, I discovered a passion for barefoot water skiing.
My older brother was a barefooter and I wanted to learn the sport.
There were no other females on Christie Lake who could skim the
water on their feet. I enjoyed spending my summer days with the
guys, going around and around the lake.

One day, I turned to cross the wake and slammed into the

water. In an instant, I went from hard of hearing to deaf. When I climbed in the boat, I couldn't hear my friends' voices. I didn't give it much thought at the time as my hearing had always fluctuated. I figured I must have had water in my ears. Then the roaring began. My brain was filled with the horrible sounds of unrelenting tinnitus. The sounds were difficult to drown out, especially during the night, when I desperately wanted to sleep to escape the noise.

The reality of being deaf didn't hit until the day I was to leave for Northern Illinois University. I was standing at the front door when I was hit with a sobering thought:

I'm deaf.

The tears began with a torrent and my mom joined in. How will you hear your teachers, she wanted to know. How was I going to cope in a big university when I'd struggled to understand the teachers at a community college the year before?

"You don't have to go," she said. "You can stay home and get a job."

I knew, deep down, if I didn't walk through that door, I'd never face life head on. I'd be taking the safe route and as much as I loved my family, it didn't look too appealing.

When we arrived on campus, I discovered I had been placed on a "Hearing Impaired" floor. I went to the front desk and protested. Rudely, I recall.

"I'm not like them," I said. "I want to be on a 'normal' floor."

Yes. I cringe just typing this. My frame of reference and my attitude at the time were nothing short of abysmal.

The Turnaround

At first, living among deaf and hard of hearing students was very much like being dropped in Japan and not knowing a shred of Japanese. The hands were waving around so fast in American Sign Language that most conversations were nothing but a blur. Some lips moved, some didn't. I learned to take refuge with those I could lipread. Here and there, a kind soul would reach out and teach me the new language.

My social life flourished on the weekends, when I discovered I could fit in pretty well after a couple of beers. However, I was struggling in my classes, straining to lipread my teachers and the students around me. The nights were lonely and in the quiet stillness, the ringing sounds would envelope the darkness. I spent night after night crying.

One morning, I had an epiphany. I was lying in bed, thinking about my life. I came to the realization that I had two choices: I could either continue to be miserable and struggle each day, or I could embrace the new path on the journey and become the best possible deaf person I could be.

I thought of the new friends I had met. Some of them couldn't utter a word verbally, yet, they were living full, vibrant, happy lives all around me.

I chose the latter.

I got out of bed and for the first time in my life, I pulled my hair in a ponytail, slapped on my hearing aid and went out in public for the first time with the device perched for all to see. I had never done that before. I felt pretty self-conscious while riding the bus–I was sure everyone was staring at me. I marched into the disability office, returned the useless FM system and asked for interpreters for every class. I lipread the interpreters and quickly began to pick up American Sign Language. By the time I graduated, I was substitute teaching in sign classes.

Life became very full. I met my husband in college and we traveled with a deaf volleyball team for 12 years. Our three kids ended up with the same gene–becoming deaf and hard of hearing at two, four and two years of age. I had various jobs over the years and life was humming along.

Fast Forward to Age 44

The email from my husband sat in my box for weeks,

unopened. As I purged my emails one by one, I almost deleted the one he sent. I took a second glance at the subject line: "Barefoot Skier Lands on Her Feet at 66."

A 66-year-old, female barefoot water skier? Intrigued, I clicked on the link. It was a TODAY show segment and the smiling face of Judy Myers filled the screen. She wasn't just smiling, she was glowing. The kind of glow you have when you're deep into your passion. The TODAY show was not captioned, but the action on screen was enough to fill me with tears. Here was a heavy-set, older woman skimming on the water, doing a sport I thought I could no longer do.

I sat paralyzed in my seat and hit the replay button again and again. My eyes took in Judy's every move on the water. The guy driving the boat was interviewed and I was able to lipread some of what he said.

Judy Myers. I Googled her name and found a Subway "Fit to Boom" segment featuring the same gal with the brilliant white teeth. The same boat driver showed up.

At 44-years-of-age, I felt old. I was overweight, out of shape and had long ago abandoned my passion for barefoot water skiing. Yet, if a 66-year old woman could barefoot water ski, well, why not me? Was there really anything stopping me from unwrapping my passion once again? I wanted to get back on the water–I wanted that look of joy I saw on Judy's face–the joy I had buried when I gave up the sport.

I sent the links to a friend and asked her to type out what was being said. I was desperate to know what they were talking about. What was this woman's story? How did she get into an extreme sport like this at the age of 53? From the typed transcript, I learned Judy tried the sport on a dare during an outing with some gal pals. "You have one shot at this," she warned her friends. Scooting out on the boom and putting her feet in the water–she found herself standing up. The experience gave her a thrill like no other. She was hooked.

Judy took up barefoot competition and struck up a friendship with Keith St. Onge, the two-time World Barefoot Champion, who turned out to be the guy driving the boat in both videos. After she retired from working at a college, Judy went to work for Keith at his ski school in Florida. I knew I had to contact her. I wanted to figure out a way to get my feet wet again. A Facebook search hit the jackpot. I sent Judy a friend request and a message with the short version of my story.

"Come down to Florida and we'll get you back on the water," she said.

In March 2010, I arrived at the World Barefoot Center in Winter Haven and met with Judy and Keith. I was a bundle of nerves. I could hardly pay attention to Keith's instructions on the dock–a tiny part of me just wanted to get up and leave. (Keith later told me he thought I was being rude!) Six of us piled into the boat and as I watched the others perform on the water–doing one foots, tumble turns and barefooting backwards–I wondered just what the heck was I doing down there. For a minute there yet again, I just wanted to climb out of the boat and go home. Everyone was so nice and encouraging.

Soon it was my turn–and the moment I put my feet on the water I felt like a teenager again. I stood up on my first try and I just wanted to do it again and again. I was out of breath and terribly out of shape, but I was hooked. Three weeks later, I was back in Florida for work and I went to the World Barefoot Center again.

Then I never left.

To say my life did a 180-degree turn that day is an understatement. I ended up becoming a sponsored skier and staff member at the World Barefoot Center, managing the blog. I took up competition at the age of 45, becoming the only deaf competitive barefoot water skier. I learned to do tricks I couldn't even fathom doing as a teen–including barefooting backwards and toe holds. Keith and I ended up writing a book together, *Gliding Soles, Lessons from a Life on Water*.

Ever since I put my feet back on the water, life has been incredible. I learned so many lessons from unwrapping my passions and now I coach others on how to live a passionate life.

Becoming deaf turned out to be a blessing. My whole world opened up after I became deaf. What I thought was the most awful thing to happen to me turned out to be a wonderful thing instead. I used to wish I could hear, thinking that life would be just dandy if only I had the full sense of hearing. There's a line from a Garth Brooks song that fits right in:

"Some of God's greatest gifts are unanswered prayers."

Now About You...

I hope you enjoyed the amazing deaf and hard of hearing people featured in this book. I certainly had a blast interviewing each of them and sharing their stories.

The possibilities today are virtually endless for deaf and hard of hearing people. Remember, you were born with certain gifts, abilities, talents and skills. It's up to you to use them, to share your passions with the world. You *will* encounter people who hold you back, people who won't believe in you and there will be times you will want to give up. Surround yourself with people who uplift you, who believe in you, and who want to see you achieve your dreams and live your passions. Find a mentor and learn from them. Above all, a passionate life comes to those who persist–and to those who do not give up their dreams, even during the hardest moments.

www.karenputz.com
karen@karenputz.com

Made in the USA
Columbia, SC
21 May 2018